MW01164813

DYSAUTONOMIA
DIARY

Essays and Tips for

Enjoying Life

Despite Chronic Illness

Hold on to hope.

By

Laura Seil Ruszczyk and

Sharon A. Roloff

We believe in you!

Foreword by Dr. Blair P. Grubb, world-renowned

dysautonomia expert and cardiologist

NFB Publishing
Buffalo, NY

Printed in the United States of America

DYSAUTONOMIA DIARY: Essays and Tips forEnjoying Life
Despite Chronic Illness/ Ruszczyk & Roloff— 1st Edition

ISBN: 979-83706869-8-6

1. Physical Impairments>Self Help
2. Stress Management Self-Help
3. Consciousness & Thought Philosophy
4. Pain Management>Books
5. Medical Neuropsychology
6. Healing
7. Chronic Pain>Books

NFB
NFB Publishing/Amelia Press
119 Dorchester Road
Buffalo, New York 14213

For more information visit Nfbpublishing.com

"You have to fight it as best you can. But at the same time you have to learn to live your life despite it; to sort of live life and enjoy what you can despite your illness."

Dr. Blair P. Grubb

DEDICATION

LAURA: To my dear family Stephen, Gerard, Sara, Ethan and Lindsay and all the angels I encounter on this journey.

SHARON: To Ed my husband, daughters and sons-in-laws: Amy Balbierz, Kate and Bret Berkey, and Lindsey Balbierz and Tom Takigayama. They are my steadfast support. And to my grandchildren Emmy, Owen and Noah, who fill my heart with the joy of exploration.

TABLE OF CONTENTS

Foreword: Dr. Blair P. Grubb

"In the middle of the road of my life
I awoke in a deep dark wood
Where the true way
Was wholly lost..."
—Dante Alighieri
The Divine Comedy (Burton Raffel).

THE PASSAGE INTO illness is an unwilling journey into another realm. Alone and abandoned with no sense of where you are, and no maps to guide you, you become a "stranger in a strange land." Even if you somehow manage (by courage and good fortune) to find your way to safety you must confront the fact that the world you once knew, the person you once were, and the very world as you once knew it are now forever changed. Somehow you must begin to construct a new life out of the remnants of what once was, making the first tentative steps into what will be.

It is a journey that each of us will someday take. Some sooner, some later. The prospect of our own eventual infirmity and mortality is so daunting that we scarcely think of it at all. That is until it comes crashing into our lives with the sudden force of the thunderbolt. The remarkable advances in health and longevity achieved in the modern era have had the consequence of leaving us both complacent and unprepared for our own inevitable confrontation with illness and despair. Health has replaced salvation as a goal of most Americans, with illness seen as a punishment for some misdeed or ill behavior. And while poor health choices may influence our risk of illness it is often a combination of random genetic and environmental factors that determine our fates. Illness comes unexpectedly and unbidden, striking without warning. One day we awaken, as the poet Dante says "in a deep dark wood where the true way is wholly lost." Thus each person who struggles with illness begins a journey through a metaphorical hell to an uncertain future. The difficult and harrowing paths through illness is often one of self-discovery, peeling away the façades of daily life to uncover those things which are of true meaning and importance. In the end experience can be transformative, and the story of the journey can serve as a guide to those who will come afterward on their own trek through the kingdom of the sick.

What follows is Laura Ruszczyk and Sharon Roloff's tale of their battles with dysautonomia, a disturbance in the body's ability to regulate critical functions necessary to maintain life itself such as heart rate, blood pressure, body temperature and bowel motility. These once mysterious disorders can render a previously healthy individual unable to perform many of the normal activities of day-to-day living. Once cloaked in mystery, the last three decades have seen an explosion in our understanding of the normal functioning of the autonomic nervous system as well as the ways in which it can go awry. Today many people who suffer from these crippling illnesses can be helped by variety of medications and devices that can help restore the body's normal balance and function. Where there was once despair there is now hope. Laura's courage and determination in the face of chronic illness is both a testament to her character as well as a guide to others who suffer from these debilitating disorders. It is a story of hope and perseverance that can serve as an example to us all.

Blair P. Grubb MD
Professor of Medicine and Pediatrics at the University of Toledo, Health Science Campus. Director of the Electrophysiology Program and the Syncope and Autonomic Disorders Clinic at the University Medical Center.

Blair P. Grubb is a native of Baltimore, Maryland and earned an undergraduate degree in Biologic Sciences from the University of Maryland (Baltimore County). He received an M.D from the Universidad Central del Este in the Dominican Republic. He completed residency training at the Greater Baltimore Medical Center where he was also chief resident. While doing a rotation in cardiology at the Johns Hopkins Hospital he became interested in cardiac electrophysiology after watching some of the first human defibrillator implants. He then completed a fellowship in cardiology and cardiac electrophysiology at the Pennsylvania State University. He is presently a professor of medicine and pediatrics at the University of Toledo,

Health Science Campus. He is also director of the Electrophysiology Program and the Syncope and Autonomic Disorders Clinic at the University Medical Center.

Dr. Grubb has authored more than 240 scientific papers, five books and 35 book chapters. He has been awarded the University of Maryland's Distinguished Alumnus Award (1994); the Northwest Ohio American Heart Associations' Legacy of Achievement Award (2001); the Medical University of Ohio's Dean's Award for teaching excellence (1996) and the Leonard Tow Humanism in Medicine Award (2006). He has been recognized as one of "Americas Top Doctors" for 15 consecutive years and one of "Americas Best Doctors" for 12 consecutive years.

In 2009, he received the University of Toledo's Distinguished University Professor award (the first physician ever to receive the honor) and received it again in 2015 (one of the few in UT's history to receive it twice). In 2015 he received the Physician of the Year Award from Dysautonomia International. He also received the "Medical Professional of the Decade" award from the British Heart Rhythm Society and Arrhythmia Alliance in 2015, as well as the University of Toledo's "Dean's Award for Career Achievement" for 2015. In 2016 he was given the Dion D. Raftopoulos/Sigma Xi Award for "Outstanding Research." He was awarded the University of Toledo's "Outstanding Research and Scholarship Award" in 2017, as well as the University's "Outstanding Contributions in Scholarship and Creative Activity Award" in 2018. He was presented with the Dysautonomia Support Network's "Revolutionary Researcher Award" in 2019.

Dr. Grubb is widely considered one of the world's leading authorities on syncope and disorders of the autonomic nervous system. His research has helped develop a whole new field of medicine _ Autonomics_ and he has pioneered many of the diagnostic and treatment modalities that are in common use today. He is a senior editor of the journal PACE and sits on the editorial boards of numerous other journals. His hobbies include writing, and he has published more than 50 essays and poems, as well as drawings and photography. Dr. Grubb's collection of essays has been published as a book entitled "The Calling." He is a survivor of renal cancer, an event that fostered his interest in promoting physician wellness. He is a member of the Union of Concerned Scientists and Physicians for Social Responsibility. He was the husband of the late Barbara Straus M.D. for 38 years and has three children: Helen, Alex and Margaret. He is currently married to Dena Eber PhD.

ACKNOWLEDGEMENTS

Laura This book would not have been possible without the support of my dear husband of 34 years Stephen. His unwavering support, even when we had no idea what was occurring medically and we had to change our life dreams, continues to provide hope to our family.

Our children Gerard, Sara, Ethan and Lindsay, I thank for their support and marvel at the empathy that they show as a result of experiencing my changing health. I am thankful for their simple acts of kindness- grabbing me a drink/blanket/ pillow when I crash and giving me grace when my attitude plunges.

Dr. Grubb I thank for first helping me to function better physically, spiritually and emotionally but also encouraging my writing and being an amazing listener.

Dr. David Deberny who is the quarterback of my medical team but also is willing to try new things or just listen and laugh with me.

Friends Deanna Reed and Karen Gowin whom I lost in 2018. They were two of my greatest encouragers and their spirit lives on.

My tutu sisters, Hamburg HopeKeepers, Wednesday red door book club, Restministries friends, mitochondria support group members and others I have met that inspire me through their own dealings with chronic illness.

My counselor Connie Gulino, LCSWR, who in addition to helping to process my medical challenges also gently encouraged me by saying more than once "how is the book coming?"

My friends, some since childhood, others new, who have had to understand that even though I may not be able to do some things that I did as a healthy person, I am still the same person. Thank you for sticking with me.

Those angels that come and go but provide guidance and love along the way.

My dear friend Sharon who encouraged and educated me when I had no idea what was occurring and for traveling this road with me.

My siblings and other relatives who watched and gave support as I lost health and then slowly regained functioning.

Former colleagues who were of great support when my body first began to revolt against me.

Dysautonomia International which provides unwavering support, education and research to those dealing with dysautonomia and their loved ones.

Lauren Stiles, president of Dysautonomia International, who has become a friend along this journey. She is funny, wicked smart and shares my zest for life, despite chronic illnesses.

God who provides me with the strength to continue this crazy medical ride.

> **Remember: "Spread love everywhere you go. Let no one ever come to you without leaving better. Be faithful in small things because it is in them that your strength lies."**
> **—Mother Teresa**

<u>Sharon</u> To God my perfect Father in heaven, His son, my brother, sometimes I forget that He is asleep in the boat (Matthew 8:23-27) when my tempests hit; and the divine spirit infused and sealed.

To my husband Edward; he truly is a gift from divine providence. His clear, calm, steady reflective endorsement is unfaltering. Our love for each other has endured challenges, which came very unexpectedly. He is my funny, bright, and reflective safeguard, my soft place to land.

To my daughters Amy Balbierz, Kate Berkey and Lindsey Balbierz who are my best gifts ever. I truly hit the jackpot when selected to be their mom. They are poised, mature, young women who have extraordinary life skills of compassion. As teens they made runs to emergency rooms with me, and learned to drive, while chauffeuring me. They have wise life insight, and value what is truly important. They give me extraordinary nonverbal cues.

To my sons-in-law Bret Berkey and Tom Takigayama, who complete my "A Team." Everywhere I turn, they present with a steadying moment, a glance, and a nod. They anticipate my weakened moments, and always lend a hand or arm to steady my faltering.

To my beautiful grandchildren Emmy and Noah, who fill my heart with the joy of exploration.

To my CNM colleagues who covered call and scheduling.

Family and friends provided meals, rides, and coffee breaks. Your active listening sustained me.

To Laura, my co-author, and friend. "There are two of us." We have moments of ridiculous adventures; a la Lucy and Ethel of I love Lucy. It has been quite a ride.

From this support flows my style: The only thing I carry is joy. The only thing I lift up is my heart.

PREFACE

Dysautonomia (noun)-An umbrella term used to describe different medical conditions that cause a deregulation of the Autonomic Nervous System (ANS). The ANS controls such body functions as heart rate, blood pressure, temperature regulation, digestion and breathing. When this system malfunctions life becomes complicated.

Laura: When you have a medical diagnosis which is less glamorous, not well-known and with fewer doctors interested in treating than other diseases or disorders, one might feel at times like a science experiment.

Can you imagine entering a cardiologist's office with hopes of finding answers and treatment only to be told you are not sick enough for him to treat? This after barely staying conscious while in the waiting room. Or watch nurse after nurse as their eyes bugged out when they see your blood pressure - which can go from high to low just by moving positions? Or how about having a nurse ask if you drove yourself to the doctor's office, and if so, do you think that was wise? (I would never drive if unsafe). And when you mention dysautonomia to some medical personnel you are asked to spell it because they have no idea how or even what it is.

Can you fathom having to travel 200 miles to receive a full autonomic nervous system evaluation because even though you live in the second largest city in your state with a huge university and teaching medical campus, there is no comprehensive autonomic testing center? Or travel 300 miles each way to your cardiologist for the same reason. And after he implants a pacemaker to treat bradycardia you realize the pacemaker representative who covers your geographical area lacks experience to adjust it properly. So you travel 600-miles roundtrip to the cardiologist whenever you need setting changes.

I never thought of these scenarios either when I began a medical journey with dysautonomia in the summer of 2010. That summer, at the age of 46, I had two episodes on my hybrid road bike in which I had to dive off the bike and into the grass, dizzy with a racing heartbeat. My doctor's office chalked it up to dehydration, but I knew differently. I could not bike the normal 15-mile rides; I was able to go five miles. I was off physically and knew it.

Life hit crises point in December 2010. After completing a sleep study on December 2, I went home and experienced the worse stomach flu I can recall. Then on December 26, after three weeks of migraines, I was unable to stand up from the couch without extraordinary effort. My limbs were heavy, and I soon learned what it felt like to become dehydrated. My heart was screaming, beating so quickly. That was the first of many experiences receiving intravenous (IV) fluids. The primary care doctor treated me and placed me on a three-week leave from work. This internist, Dr. David Deberny of Quaker Medical Associates, Orchard Park, NY., has been with me on this entire journey and has been a critical member of my medical team. His retired partner, Dr. Francis Mezzadri, was also helpful in my treatment, having been the first medical professional to suspect an autonomic nervous system disorder and ordering a Tile Table Test (TTT).

My health spiraled out of control; I continued working but often would lie down during the day, leave early or arrive late. The few people who knew something was terribly wrong kept an eye on me when I left the bathroom as that is when I felt the weakest. This was most likely due to frequent diarrhea. After meeting the cardiologist who would dismiss me in April 2011 because I was not "sick enough," I posted this Facebook status: "I hate rollercoasters." This simple statement changed my life.

A friend private messaged me and asked if I had been on a rollercoaster. I explained that the rollercoaster was a metaphor for the crazy medical journey thus far. This friend mentioned her sister-in-law in Ohio who had the same diagnosis (at this time it was believed I had dysautonomia, but I had not undergone full autonomic testing). I was introduced to the sister-in-law via the internet and in person a few weeks later when she visited New York. Eleven years later, Sharon Roloff and I have been through many adventures together. She is a confident, trusted friend and as her brother so eloquently stated "there are two of you."

I wish Sharon did not share this diagnosis. And I surmise many who read our book are people with a dysautonomia diagnosis or another chronic condition, or those who love them. But hopefully medical students/professionals who seek a better grasp of some of the physical, emotional and spiritual aspects of this unpredictable diagnosis will find our book informative. Perhaps the book will inspire medical personnel to conduct research for better treatment options or outcomes. We deserve improved treatment as do future generations. No one should have to live with the feeling that they could pass out at any moment; that their autonomic nervous system is so skewed that anything can happen. Our guts explode, our bodies don't handle temperature changes, we can't stand for very long - how odd is that?

But back to this journey. After meeting Sharon, a bond was instantly formed. We often talk, text or communicate on social media. She knows more about me than most. Early on when I was failing health wise, she supported and helped me secure an appointment with her neurologist. And this book was born, as I began journaling experiences and asked Sharon to co-author. Sharon is the brains while I am the writer. She is the former nurse practitioner who understands the medical complexities while I am the retired school counselor who began a professional life as an editor of a weekly newspaper. Writing has always fed my soul.

Realizing Sharon wasn't writing consistently, I asked her to perform two tasks: to find quotes and create tips for the book. To not confuse the reader, any piece written by Sharon (except tips) will have her initials at the end - SAR. The remainder of the book is my writing. We are equals in this process and our goal is to raise awareness of dysautonomia. Everyone's journey with dysautonomia is different with varied degrees of severity. However, we share a common bond; one of chronic illness but also chronic hope.

This is not a medical book, and it is highly personal. We hope you will find value in reading of this journey. My writing on dysautonomia continues and this book is the beginning of that journey.

Dysautonomia Diary: Essays and Tips for Enjoying Life Despite Chronic Illness is comprised of eight chapters. The book is not in chronological order, rather it is organized by topics. There will inevitably be grammatical errors in the book, which will frustrate me incredibly when I see them. However, if I wait until the book is perfect, it will never go to print.

One last point; there is ongoing research and hopefully this will result in better treatment of dysautonomia and an eventual cure. Dysautonomia International has been an invaluable lifeline for our community; providing support but also money to conduct medical studies. The nonprofit organization is also helping in the research on COVID 19 longhaulers as some are getting diagnosed with a form of dysautonomia. It is believed that the coronavirus has caused dysautonomia in these people. That is interesting, as many of us prior to the pandemic also became sick after an infection.

In addition, doctors have varied thoughts about diagnosis and treatment. When I started this journey, I was diagnosed with Postural Orthostatic Tachycardia Syndrome despite having bradycardia. Later, my cardiologist when asked about my diagnosis, mentioned Pure Autonomic Failure. I've also added several diagnoses and we are not sure which came first. These include Sjogren's syndrome, mitochondria myopathy, Ehlers Danlos syndrome, hypothyroidism, autonomic neuropathy/small fiber neuropathy, pancreatitis and migraines. Regardless of these diagnoses, my medical team and I work to provide the best quality of life I can experience. This is my prayer for all on this medical road. God bless you on your journey.

Sharon: It is ironic that I am writing a book. My high school grades were not stellar, yet I aced New York State Regents exams. My learning curve was curious. I started college without the ability to compose a theme. My English instructor started me out building a paragraph.

It is surprising that I earned two graduate degrees, the first in pediatric primary care nursing and the second in nurse midwifery. It was not until I was reading about how children learn that I realized I am a visual learner. My auditory processing, especially numbers such as drug doses, get tangled up. When I worked in intensive care units, I made laminated index cards with standard dosing of resuscitation drugs. I would watch and anticipate what was ordered. I kept these cards with me and referred to them during each code.

The following collection of vignettes came about after my symptoms worsened in 2000 at the age of 50. It is a struggle for me to document because when reviewing journals, I was painfully aware of the paradox of others' disbelief of my problems and the depth of my limitations. I could not make this stuff up. I had to retire to disability from working full time, in a faculty practice as a certified nurse midwife. I had just made a final graduate student loan payment. My entire career was about assisting mothers and children attain and maintain their highest level of wellness (thank you Dean Dr. Rozella Schlotfeldt, nurse theorist). God "got me back" by forcing me to study the endocrine and neurological systems and medical/surgical nursing in general. Irony does not even begin to describe my life.

My wish is that each health care provider considers every faint serious. My second hope, for those with this disorder, is to eventually see yourself as a new, vital light-emitting beacon. You will first realize what you do not have, before understanding what you do have. For me, giving my medical problems a name/diagnosis was a huge validation. After you stabilize, remember to help others; listen and reassure. Continue to transform into the new you.

After all, I who cannot process audible information am now an author. Who would have imagined? I encourage you to seek the truth about how your body works. To the rude and arrogant people you encounter stay poised, assured that you possess the truth.

I rely on the last words of Christ crucified:

> *Father forgive them, for they know but what they do.* (Luke 23:46)
>
> *Father into Your hands, I commend my spirit.* (Luke 23:46)
>
> *I thirst.* (John 19:28)

* Laura's medical team includes: Dr. Julian Ambrus Jr., immunologist; Dr. Michael Anzalone and Dr. Richard Habermehl, chiropractors; Dr. James Corasanti and Katherine Shanahan, PA-C, gastroenterology; Dr. William Crossetta, dentist; Dr. David Deberny, internist; Dr. Jon Dusse, ophthalmologist; Terry Eagan, physical therapist; Dr. Blair Grubb and Beverly Karabin, RN, PhD, CNP, cardiology; Constance Gulino, LCSWR, therapist; Dr. Steven Horn, cardiologist; Dr. Jenna O'Neill and Anna Roberts, P.A., dermatology; Dr. Irene Perillo, pulmonologist; Dr. Andrew Stoeckl, orthopaedic surgeon; Dr. Julie Szumigala, gynecologist; Dr. Robert Wilson and Emily Silberman, CNP, neurology.

Sharon's medical team includes: Dr. Dale Baur, oral and maxillofacial surgery; Dr. Robert Hostoffer, allergist/immunologist; Dr. Michael Koehler, gastroenterologist; Dr. Zuhayr Madhun, endocrinologist; Dr. Jeffrey Parks, surgeon; Dr. Chad Raymond, cardiologist; Dr. Thomas Stokkermans, optometrist.

When you find a group of caring physicians and medical professionals who understand or are willing to learn about dysautonomia, try to hold on to them. They are invaluable.

Introduction

A general understanding of dysautonomia will assist the reader in realizing what someone with autonomic nervous system dysfunction experiences. A roller coaster metaphor is appropriate as our days have massive ups and downs and most often there is no set pattern of predictability. Thankfully with proper medical treatment, exercise, fluids, prayer (we believe) and other self-help mechanisms a better quality of life is often possible. But by no means is this treatment plan easy; and every single day dysautonomia will rear its head. Note that research is ongoing and there are additional forms of dysautonomia and information. This is a basic primer. Most information was taken from Dysautonomia International. You can read more at **dysautonomiainternational.org**.

Definitions

WHAT IS DYSAUTONOMIA?

"Dysautonomia is an umbrella term used to describe several different medical conditions that cause a malfunction of the Autonomic Nervous System. (ANS). The autonomic nervous system controls the "automatic" functions of the body that we do not consciously think about including heart rate, blood pressure, digestion, pupil dilation and constriction, kidney function and temperature regulation. People living with various forms of dysautonomia have trouble regulating these systems. This may result in lightheadedness, fainting, unstable blood pressure, abnormal heart rates, malnutrition, headaches, fatigue and other symptoms.

Dysautonomia is not rare. More than 70 million people worldwide live with various forms of this disorder. This number is increasing as doctors are seeing more cases of COVID-19 long haulers that are diagnosed with dysautonomia. Research is expanding and these numbers are expected to rise. People of any age, gender or race can be impacted. There is currently no cure for any form of dysautonomia, but research continues. Despite the high prevalence of dysautonomia, most patients take years to be diagnosed due to a lack of awareness amongst the public and within the medical profession.

BASICS OF THE AUTONOMIC NERVOUS SYSTEM

The autonomic nervous system (ANS) is a very complex system of nerves in the brain, spinal cord, and peripheral nerves that reach out to the limbs and organs. The ANS can be divided into three main areas. The central (brain) portions of the ANS are found in the medulla oblongata in the lower brain stem and in the hypothalamus. The other two portions of the ANS are found in the peripheral nerves, including the sympathetic nervous system branch, and the parasympathetic nervous system branch. The medulla oblongata is a part of the brain that regulates cardiac, respiratory and vasomotor control along with reflexes like coughing, sneezing, vomiting and swallowing. The hypothalamus, another part of the brain, performs a supporting role by linking the nervous system to the endocrine system. The hypothalamus regulates body temperature, thirst, hunger, sleep and circadian rhythms in the body. Through endocrine control, the hypothalamus also plays a role in regulating blood volume and blood pressure.

The sympathetic nervous system is commonly associated with the "fight or flight" responses - those bodily reactions that you need to quickly respond in an emergency. When faced with a life-threatening situation, our human instinct takes over and we either fight the danger we are facing or take flight and run from danger. The sympathetic nervous system allows the body to do this rapidly. For example, in the face of danger the sympathetic nervous system will cause bronchial dilation - this allows the person to breathe better while fighting or running away from the situation. Likewise, the heart will beat stronger and faster, also prepping the body to fight or flight.

The parasympathetic nervous system is commonly associated with the "rest and digest" responses - those bodily actions needed to restore energy and rest the body. For example, chewing food triggers the parasympathetic nervous system to increase production of saliva and digestion in the gut. The parasympathetic nervous system also increases gallbladder function, which assists in the digestive process.

Some common forms of dysautonomia include:

Postural Orthostatic Tachycardia Syndrome (POTS); Neurocardiogenic Syncope (NCS); Pure Autonomic Failure (PAF) and Multiple System Atrophy (MSA).

POSTURAL ORTHOSTATIC TACHYCARDIA SYNDROME

POTS is a form of dysautonomia that is associated with the presence of excessive tachycardia and other symptoms upon standing. POTS predominantly impacts young women who look healthy on the outside, but POTS can affect anyone at any age. About 25 percent of POTS patients are disabled and unable to work. POTS is estimated to impact between one and three million Americans, and millions more worldwide. This number is increasing as of 2022 due to post COVID long haulers that are being diagnosed with POTS and other forms of dysautonomia. POTS is a chronic condition.

DIAGNOSTIC CRITERIA

The current diagnostic criterion for POTS is a heart rate increase of 30 beats per minute (bpm) or more, or over 120 bpm, within the first 10 minutes of standing. In children and adolescents, a standard of 40 bpm or more increase has been adopted. POTS is often diagnosed by a Tilt Table Test. If such testing is unavailable, POTS can be diagnosed with bedside measurements of heart rate and blood pressure taken in the supine (laying down) and standing up position at two, five and 10-minute intervals. Doctors may perform more detailed tests to evaluate the autonomic nervous system in POTS patients, such as Quantitative Sudomotor Axon Reflex Test (QSART), Thermoregulatory Sweat Test (TST), small fiber skin biopsies, gastric motility studies and more.

SIGNS AND SYMPTOMS

While the diagnostic criteria focus on the abnormal heart rate increase upon standing, POTS usually presents with symptoms much more complex. POTS patients often have hypovolemia (low blood volume) and high levels of plasma norepinephrine while standing. About half of POTS patients have a small fiber neuropathy that impacts their sudomotor nerves. Many POTS patients also experience fatigue, headaches, lightheadedness, heart palpitations, exercise intolerance, nausea, diminished concentration, syncope (fainting), coldness or pain in the extremities, chest pain and shortness of breath. Patients can develop a reddish-purple color in the legs upon standing, believed to be caused by blood pooling or poor circulation. The color change subsides upon returning to a reclined position.

PROGNOSIS

Some patients have mild symptoms and can continue with normal work, school, social and recreational activities. For others, symptoms may be so severe that normal life activities, such as bathing, housework, eating, sitting upright, walking or standing can be significantly limited.

POTS CLASSIFICATIONS

POTS researchers have classified POTS in various ways. Dr. Blair Grubb has described POTS as "primary" or "secondary." "Primary" refers to POTS with no other identifiable medical condition. "Secondary" refers to POTS with the presence of another medical condition known to cause or contribute to POTS symptoms. Dr. Julian Stewart has described "high flow" and "low flow" POTS, based upon the flow of blood in the patients' lower limbs.

Other researchers have described POTS based on some of its more prominent characteristics: hypovolemic POTS, which is associated with low blood volume; partial dysautonomia or neuropathic POTS which is associated with a partial autonomic neuropathy; and hyperadrenergic POTS which is associated with elevated levels of norepinephrine. These are not distinct medical conditions and many POTS patients have two or three of the different characteristics present.

WHO DEVELOPS POTS?

POTS can strike any age, gender, or race, but it is often seen in women of childbearing age (between the ages of 15 and 50). Men and boys can develop it as well, but approximately 80 percent of patients are female. POTS is not caused by anxiety. POTS patients are often misdiagnosed with having an anxiety or panic disorder. However, people with POTS have real, physical symptoms. Research has shown that POTS patients are similarly or even less likely to suffer from anxiety or panic disorders than the general population.

WHAT CAUSES POTS?

POTS is a heterogeneous group of disorders with similar clinical magnifications. POTS is not a disease, rather it is a cluster of symptoms that are frequently seen together. It is often difficult to discover what has caused POTS in each person. While research is trying to figure out the root cause of POTS there are several underlying conditions and diseases that are known to be associated with POTS. A partial list includes: autoimmune diseases such as sjogren's syndrome, lupus, autoimmune autonomic ganglionopathy and sarcoidosis; chiari malformation; delta storage pool deficiency; diabetes and pre-diabetes; Ehlers Danlos Syndrome; genetic disorders; infections such as mononucleosis, COVID-19; and Epstein Barr virus; lyme disease; multiple sclerosis; mitochondrial diseases, mast cell activation disorders, traumas and more.

TREATMENT

Each patient is different, thus consulting with a physician who has experience in treating autonomic disorders is important. (Dysautonomia International has a doctor recommendation list which can be found on its web site dysautonomiainternational.org). The most common treatments for POTS include increasing fluid intake to two to three liters per day; increasing salt consumption to between 3,000 and 10,000 mg per day; wearing compression stockings or compression wear; raising the head of the bed (to conserve blood volume); performing reclined exercises such as rowing, recumbent bicycling, and swimming;

eating small meals and a healthy diet and avoiding sub-stances and situations that worsen orthostatic symptoms. There are several medications that may help symptoms. These may include Midodrine, Fludrocortisone, Propran-olol, Pyridostigmine and Ivabradines. Each person reacts differently to medications and may need to try several before improvement is noted. If an underlying cause of POTS is discerned, it is important to treat the cause. There is currently no cure for POTS. Researchers, however, be-lieve some patients will see improvements over time.

SYNCOPE

Syncope is the formal medical term for fainting, de-scribing a temporary loss of consciousness due to a sudden decline in blood flow to the brain. Syncope can be caused by numerous things. Some forms of syncope are benign, while other forms can indicate serious health problems. After a syncopal episode, an individual may be temporar-ily unconscious, but will revive and slowly return to nor-mal. Syncope can occur in otherwise healthy people and affects all age groups but occurs more often in the elderly.

Syncope accounts for approximately three percent of emergency room visits and six percent of hospital admis-sions. It is important to distinguish syncope from "dizzi-ness" or "pre-syncope," which generally refers to an alter-ation in balance, vision, or perception of the environment, without the loss of consciousness.

TYPES OF SYNCOPE

NEUROCARDIOGENIC SYNCOPE (NCS) is the most common form of dysautonomia. It is a temporary loss of consciousness associated with a drop in blood pressure quickly followed by a slowed heart rate. Some individuals with NCS have a mild case, with fainting spells once or twice in their lifetime. However, other individuals have severe NCS which results in fainting several times per day. This can lead to falls, broken bones and even traumatic brain injury. Individuals with moderate to severe NCS have difficulty engaging in work, school and social activities due to the frequent fainting attacks. The low blood pressure leads to syncope if it is severe enough, or to light-headedness (pre-syncope) if less severe or if the patient is lying down. There is general agreement among medical experts that these symptoms are due to changes in heart rate and blood pressure. NCS is also known by Neurally Mediated Syncope and Neurally Mediated Hypotension.

REFLEX SYNCOPE is sometimes known as "the common faint" because it is somewhat common. It can occur for a variety of reasons, usually termed "trigger events." Estimates of isolated fainting episodes range from 15 to 25 percent in young people. About 25 percent of elderly people faint, which may relate to use of medications or to physiological changes. The overall lifetime incidence of fainting can approach 50 percent.

REFLEX SYNCOPE INCLUDES:

- Vasovagal Syncope. Trigger events include emotional stress, trauma, the sight of blood or needles, prolonged standing and sudden fear.
- Carotid Sinus Syncope. This occurs because of constriction of the carotid artery in the neck. It can occur after turning the head, while shaving, or when wearing a tight collar.
- Situational Syncope. Occurs during or immediately after urination, defecation, coughing, laughing, or because of gastrointestinal stimulation.

CARDIAC SYNCOPE/HEART-RHYTHM DISORDERS may cause syncope if the heart rate is too slow or too fast, but variable. Occasionally, heart-rhythm problems cause syncope in otherwise healthy people, but individuals with underlying heart disease (such as a previous heart attack or heart valve disease) are at greater risk. Cardiac syncope is often quite serious. The first step in evaluating syncope is to evaluate the patient for possible cardiac syncope.

CAUSES OF CARDIAC SYNCOPE MAY INCLUDE:

- Long QT syndrome. An electrical heart abnormality that can produce dangerous arrhythmias.
- Arrhythmogenic Right Ventricle Dysplasia (ARVD). A rare form of cardiomyopathy in which the heart muscle of the right ventricle is replaced by fat and/or fibrous tissue. The right ventricle is dilated and contracts poorly. As a result, the ability of the heart to pump blood is usually weakened.

- Cardiomyopathies. Diseases of the heart muscle.
- Left Ventricular Outflow Obstruction. Encompasses a series of stenotic lesions starting in the anatomic left ventricular outflow tract and stretching to the descending portion of the aortic arch.
- Myocardial Infarction. Heart attack.
- Primary Pulmonary Hypertension. A rare disease characterized by elevated pulmonary artery pressure with no apparent cause.
- Heart Arrhythmias such as ventricular tachycardia (fast heart rate), bradycardia (very slow heart rate) and related arrhythmic events.

DIAGNOSTIC CRITERIA AND TREATMENT

The diagnosis of syncope often focuses on ruling out potentially serious causes of syncope, particularly heart-related problems. Tests include extensive medical history; electrocardiogram (EKG); orthostatic vitals; echocardiogram (ECG); cardiac exercise stress test; blood tests; and Tilt Table Test. Treatment includes: avoiding syncope triggers; increasing salt and fluid intake; wearing compression stockings and garments; mild aerobic conditioning and medications. Medications may include beta-blockers, SSRIs, Midodrine and Disopyramide.

PROGNOSIS

The prognosis for syncope patients depends on which type of syncope is present. Patients and caregivers must be educated on what to do during a syncopal attack and how to minimize the chance of injury. In most cases, the patient should be gently placed in a reclined position, and if possible, the feet elevated. Consult with a doctor on what to do during or after a syncopal episode, based on the type of syncope you or your loved one has been diagnosed with. Most patients will improve with proper education on the avoidance of triggers, supplementary hydration, and in some cases, medication.

PURE AUTONOMIC FAILURE (PAF)

Pure autonomic failure is a peripheral degenerative disorder of the autonomic nervous system. PAF was formerly known as Bradbury-Eggleston Syndrome, after the two researchers who first described it in 1925. PAF is also referred to as idiopathic orthostatic hypotension by some physicians. PAF is one of three diseases classified as a primary autonomic disorder. The other two are multiple system atrophy and Parkinson's Disease.

DIAGNOSIS CRITERIA

The definitive diagnosis of hypotension as the cause of orthostatic symptoms is usually made by the demonstration of a decline in systolic blood pressure of 20 mm Hg and diastolic blood pressure of 10 mm Hg after at least one minute of standing. However, a decrease in systolic blood pressure by 50 mm HG or greater is not unusual. Several readings should be taken. PAF patients have greatly reduced catecholamine levels. These levels are very low while lying down and have little increase upon standing.

Plasma and urinary norepinephrine levels are usually greatly reduced. These indicators help diagnose PAF.

SYMPTOMS

PAF usually affects more men than women, in middle to later life. However, it is occasionally seen in younger patients. PAF is characterized by orthostatic hypotension (low blood pressure upon standing), a low resting supine plasma noradrenaline concentration that does not increase significantly upon standing, a decreased ability to sweat, persistent neck pain that is often relieved when lying down, raised blood pressure while laying down, changes in urinary habits, and poor tolerance of high altitude. In men with PAF, impotence often occurs. Researchers are unsure what causes PAF, but in some cases a loss of nerve cells in the spinal cord has been documented.

TREATMENT

Treatment often focuses on counteracting the effects of orthostatic hypotension, and supine hypertension, which can be difficult. Patients are routinely advised to increase fluid and salt intake, wear compression garments, sleep with the head of their bed at an upright angle, and medications as directed by a physician.

PROGNOSIS

The prognosis is good for PAF compared to other similar disorders, such as Multiple System Atrophy, with a slower progression and more lifestyle and pharmacological treatment options. Most PAF patients survive 20 years or more after diagnosis, many into their 80's. The cause of death is often recurrent infection or a pulmonary embolism. PAF patients have a reduced risk of heart attacks and stroke.

MULTIPLE SYSTEM ATROPHY (MSA)

MSA is a fatal form of dysautonomia. It is a neurodegenerative disorder with some similarities to Parkinson's disease. Unlike Parkinson's patients, MSA patients usually become fully bedridden within two years of diagnosis and die within five-10 years. MSA is considered a rare disease, with an estimated 350,000 patients worldwide. MSA patients have more widespread autonomic nerve damage than typical Parkinson's patients. Since MSA can cause widespread nerve damage, it may cause diverse symptoms throughout the body.

Physicians often classify MSA as either MSA-P or MSA-C. MSA-P patients have predominantly Parkinson-like symptoms: tremors, muscle rigidity and slowness of voluntary movements. MSA-C patients predominantly show signs of cerebellar dysfunction: gait and limb ataxia (ataxia being a lack of control of muscle movements).

DIAGNOSTIC CRITERIA

MSA can be a challenge to diagnose. MSA is frequently confused with Parkinson's Disease, Pure Autonomic Failure (PAF), or Progressive Supranuclear Palsy. The top practitioners and researchers in the field have prepared a consensus statement on the diagnosis of Multiple System

Atrophy. The work-up may include autonomic testing, EMG testing, blood tests, sleep studies, catecholamine testing, and biopsies. Often, MSA can only be confirmed during an autopsy.

SYMPTOMS

Not every patient has each symptom of MSA. Some early symptoms of MSA may include: neurogenic orthostatic hypotension (a drop in blood pressure upon standing that can result in lightheadedness, dizziness and even fainting); headaches; dry eyes, mouth and skin; abnormally dilated pupils; impotence and loss of bladder control.

Some of the later stage symptoms may include sleep apnea: stridor (a loud noise during inhalation); heart arrhythmias; difficulty eating, swallowing or chewing food; difficulty speaking; monotone voice, low volume of voice and slow speaking.

Symptoms that may be seen at varying times during the course of the illness: unusual or reduced ability to make facial expressions; staring with the eyes; loss of fine motor skills; muscle aches and rigidity; loss of balance; movement difficulties; difficulty sleeping; cognitive impairment; loss of bowel control; loss of sweating in areas of the body; nausea; difficulty digesting foods; unstable or stooped/slumped posture; unsteady gait; difficulty bending arms and legs; difficulty starting any voluntary movement; tremors, which may worsen with excitement, stress, or fatigue; finger-thumb rubbing; vision changes, decreased or blurry vision; confusion: dementia and depression.

WHO DEVELOPS MSA?

MSA is most often seen in persons over the age of 50, with a slightly higher incidence in men. However, women and younger patients can develop it. Estimates are that approximately 25,000 to 100,000 Americans have MSA at any given time. It is not known what causes this. Research is ongoing.

TREATMENT

There is currently no cure for MSA and no treatments proven to slow the neurological degeneration. However, there are treatments to help manage some of the symptoms, and to help the patient live the fullest life possible. Current therapeutic strategies are primarily based on dopamine replacement and improvement of autonomic failure. Physicians may prescribe medications to help control the patient's blood pressure, gastric motility, sleeping difficulties, tremors, depression, pain and other symptoms.

PROGNOSIS

MSA typically progresses rapidly over a period of seven to 10 years, with the mean survival rate of 9.3 years from the time of the first symptoms. About 80 percent of patients are disabled within five years of the onset of motor symptoms. It is estimated that only 20 percent of MSA patients survive beyond 12 years. Patients continue to experience neurological degeneration until they lose motor skills, become confined to bed, and eventually die. Many MSA patients succumb to pneumonia and other respiratory infections, choking or cardiac arrest. MSA does not go into remission and there is currently no cure. There are considerable genetic research and clinical investigations taking place to improve quality of life and treatment options for MSA patients.

Dysautonomia can also occur secondary to other medical conditions, such as diabetes, multiple sclerosis, rheumatoid arthritis, celiac disease, Sjogren's syndrome, lupus, mast cell activation disorder, mitochondrial myopathy and Parkinson's disease. There is currently no cure for dysautonomia, but secondary forms may improve with treatment of the underlying disease. There are some treatments available to improve quality of life, both with medications and lifestyle changes/adaptations. Even using all treatments available, many dysautonomia patients experience disabling symptoms that significantly reduce their quality of life.

ADDITIONAL FORMS OF DYSAUTONOMIA INCLUDE:

AUTONOMIC DYSREFLEXIA. Autonomic Dysreflexia (AD) is a form of autonomic dysfunction associated with spinal cord injuries. When an AD attack occurs, there is an irritant impacting the person below the level of their spinal cord injury. Because their autonomic nervous system cannot process messages properly, this results in a severe spike in blood pressure, flushing above the spinal injury, nasal stuffiness and other symptoms. AD is serious and can lead to a stroke if not treated properly during an attack.

BAROREFLEX FAILURE. The baroreceptor reflex, or baroreflex, is one of the body's homeostatic mechanisms for maintaining blood pressure. If the baroreceptor itself or part of its messaging system fails, this is referred to as baroreflex failure. Patients often deal with normal or low resting blood pressure and very high or volatile blood pressure during periods of stress.

CEREBRAL SALT WASTING SYNDROME. Cerebral salt-wasting syndrome (CSWS) is a rare condition featuring hyponatremia and dehydration in response to a physical injury or the presence of tumors in or surrounding the brain. The hyponatremia is due to excessive sodium excretion from the kidney resulting from a centrally mediated process.

DIABETIC AUTONOMIC NEUROPATHY. Diabetic autonomic neuropathy is a secondary form of autonomic dysfunction, but it is likely the most common form of autonomic dysfunction in the world. An estimated 20 percent of all diabetics suffer from diabetic autonomic neuropathy, which equates to about 69 million people worldwide. This is a serious complication of diabetes associated with an increased risk of cardiovascular mortality.

FAMILIAL DYSAUTONOMIA. Familial dysautonomia (FD) is an exceptionally rare genetic disorder seen almost entirely in persons of Ashkenazi Jewish descent. There are only about 350 people worldwide living with this disease. FD is very serious and is considered fatal, although with better treatments, patients are living longer than they did in the past.

REFLEX SYMPATHETIC DYSTROPHY (Complex Regional Pain Syndrome). Reflex Sympathetic Dystrophy is an extremely painful neurological condition. Some doctors consider it a form of dysautonomia, while others disagree."

AUTONOMIC TESTING (taken from uhhospitals.com)

Autonomic testing is a noninvasive diagnostic examination of the nerves that regulate different functions of the body.

The Autonomic Screen is used to test the nerves that control heart rate, blood pressure and sweat glands. This screen has four noninvasive tests, heart rate deep breathing, Valsalva maneuver, tilt table testing, and quantitative sudomotor axon reflex test.

The Reflex Sympathetic Dystrophy/Chronic Regional Pain Syndrome Screen (RSD) is used to test the nerves that control skin temperature, skin blood flow, limb volume, sweat glands, and muscle blood flow. This screen has nine different noninvasive components to the test.

The Quantitative Sensory Test Screen (QST) is used to test the nerves that sense vibration, heat, and cooling. This screen has six different noninvasive components.

The Thermoregulatory Sweat Test Screen (TST) is used to test nerves that control the sweat glands all over the body. This test is used in conjunction with the ANS screen, by the referring physician.

Cardiovascular Autonomic Tests assess autonomic control of heart rate and blood pressure. Your blood pressure will be measured using a standard blood pressure cuff on one arm, and a small device that measures blood pressure continuously on your finger. To measure your heart rate, you will have cardiac leads placed on your chest and attached to an electrocardiogram (EKG). During the first test you will take slow deep breaths consecutively for a minute. Your heart rate and blood pressure will be measured and analyzed by a computer program. The purpose of the test is to measure heart rate variability.

The next test will require you to blow into a mouthpiece against resistance. Again, your heart rate and blood pressure will be measured and analyzed by a computer program. This test is also designed to measure heart rate and blood pressure variability.

The third test is the **Tilt Table Test** (TTT). During the TTT the patient is on a motorized table, which will take you slowly from a lying to a standing position. You will stand at a 70-degree angle for about 20 to 40 minutes (less time if you pass out) with your heart rate and blood pressure monitored and recorded. The purpose of the TTT is to determine whether you experience any changes in your heart rate or blood pressure upon a change in position. During the TTT some patients may faint. A technician is present, and you are continuously monitored. The cardiovascular autonomic tests generally take one and a half hours to complete.

Quantitative Sudomotor Axon Reflex Test (QSART) will test the function of your sweat glands, which are under autonomic control. The QSART is very useful in determining whether there is damage to the small nerves that control your sweat glands, and whether that is contributing to an autonomic disorder. During the QSART, your sweat glands will be stimulated using a small electrical current. The electrical stimulation will allow acetylcholine, a chemical naturally found in the body, to reach and activate the sweat glands. Once stimulated, your sweat glands will sweat, and the amount of sweat produced will be analyzed with a computer program. This test will be done on one side of your body in four sites, including the forearm, hand, leg and foot. Your shoe and sock on the appropriate leg will be removed and skin will then be cleaned using acetone. Capsules designed to hold the acetylcholine will be snugly attached to you in the four appropriate locations. The current will then be turned on and will remain on for five minutes during which sweat responses are measured. The total time for this test is approximately 30 minutes. During the test, you may experience moderate burning or tingling sensation.

Quantitative Sensory Test (QST) is used to assess your response to vibration and temperature sensations. The QST is helpful in assessing whether you have experienced nerve damage. The test will require you to remove your shoes and socks. A small device will then be used to administer a small vibration or temperature change. You must indicate whether or not you felt the stimulus. The QST uses a computer program to measure and analyze responses. During the test, you will feel mild vibrations and hot and cold sensations. You should experience little or no discomfort during this test. This set of testing usually takes approximately one hour.

Thermoregulatory Sweat Test (TST) is a test that evaluates your entire body's ability to sweat. The thermoregulatory sweat test is an important diagnostic tool for physicians in identifying and differentiating between many neurological disorders because it assesses your entire body's response to heat. You will be required to wear a disposable bathing suit for this test. You will then lie on a table while the technician applies a powder to cover the entire front of the body. This powder is designed to change color when it becomes wet. After administration of the powder, four capsules will be snugly attached to the forearm, hand, leg and foot to collect the sweat you produce while in the heating box. You will then enter the heated glass box where you will remain for up to 30 minutes. During this time, your body temperature and sweat production will be closely observed. You will be monitored very closely. You may feel uncomfortable due to the powder and the heat. The powder on your skin will turn from an orange to a purple color when it becomes wet, indicating areas where you did or did not sweat. At the conclusion of the test, you will be slowly removed from the heating box, giving the body time to adjust to the changes in temperature. Your picture will then be taken as part of the medical record. This picture will be used to generate a report showing where you did or did not sweat. Following the test, you will take a shower to wash off the remaining powder. This test takes about two hours.

RULING IN/RULING OUT: THE QUEST FOR ANSWERS

Look up at the sky on a clear night. There are many stars to view; and it seems there are just as many medical tests we undergo. It is not about a single star (or test) that is not twinkling brightly. It is about a constellation, which forms a pattern of results. This is a tedious process but clarifies a diagnosis. Do not obsess about each result. It may take years to sort out the source of your health problems; for many of us the treatment plan is focused on managing symptoms.

There are many reasons why we have vascular collapse, or syncope. The examiner must focus through the telescope at the big picture. All the major systems orchestrate how the body functions. Hormones are the tiny chemicals that work at junctions, nerves, muscles, food delivery and storage, and blood flow. The heart, an amazing electrical pump, is explored if the brain does not get enough oxygen to stay conscious.

Above all, do not panic from the implications of each test. The first approach doctors take is to eliminate the more common diagnoses. You will have various blood draws. To do your part, help your veins become more prominent by performing bicep curls. Wrap your arm in a heating pad. This helps especially if you are cold. Lie down. Tell the phlebotomist that you have "a vagal response," which is a fainting reflex. If you pass out, fall and get hurt, there will be an incident report. The phlebotomist will want to avoid the faint.

Some parts of the work up are unpleasant. I always saw

this on a continuum, from not too bad to confining, to when will this be over, to no way, never again.

Magnetic Resonance Imaging (MRI) can be claustrophobic; your head goes into this birdcage contraption, and you are fastened to a sliding platform. I ask the technician to tell me when it is half and then three quarters complete, so that I can mentally prepare.

Autonomic testing is typically done off your medications. It evokes the same physiological responses of abrupt changes in gravity. The Tilt Table Test (TTT) is the most common of these tests. During the TTT, you lie down and are strapped to a table. The table is then elevated 70 degrees upright. Leg or foot movement is restricted so that the patient cannot compensate for changing vital signs. The technician monitors vitals and you report symptoms. If you pass out you will be lowered to a lying position and assisted. Caution: vomiting can be induced. When test is completed, ask for a copy of your TTT results with heartbeat and blood pressure readings cited throughout.

I am a board-certified chicken; this is my comfort:

It is the Lord who goes before you; he will be with you and will never fail you or forsake you. So do not fear or be dismayed. (Deuteronomy 31:8)

Come to me you who labor and are overburdened, and I will give you rest. Shoulder my yoke and learn from me; for I am gentle and humble in heart, and you will find rest for your souls. (Matthew 11:28-30)

These versus are put to music in "Be Not Afraid" by Scott Weiland: I go before you always, come follow me, and I will give you rest. SAR

MANY SYMPTOMS MAY EQUAL MULTIPLE DIAGNOSES

If it walks like a duck, is it a duck? Symptoms like bloating, fainting, racing heart beats and reactions to sparkly lights bring referrals to those who specialize in gastrointestinal, neurological, heart or eye disorders. Specialists take years of study, reading, and client exposure to master their field of ducks.

When doctors prioritize the solving of the mystery, the tendency is to take the most common explanation, description and diagnosis. It becomes very difficult, because we are not the rule (duck), but rather the exception. We are the zebra. We carry unique stripes and must be looked at differently.

We present with a myriad of symptoms, some more dominant than others. Furthermore, when nothing appears to be physically wrong, we are ascribed an emotional label: anxious, depressed, conversional and obsessively focused.

Since my earliest exposure to a dysautonomia support group, there were several curious observations. Most participants carried a dual diagnosis. These may include Hashimoto's thyroiditis, gastroparesis, migraines, Sjogren's syndrome, diabetes, multiple system atrophy, Ehlers-Danlos syndrome, idiopathic anaphylaxis, mitochondrial myopathy, mast cell activation disorder and others. Co-morbidities are partnered diagnoses.

The second thread I observed was a pattern of insult in the form of a trauma: an elective surgery, concussion, motor vehicle accident, or an infection which tripped the switch sending the person in to autonomic dysfunction. We are all asked, "when did this start?"

A third curiosity is that there were many who worked in public exposure occupations: nurses, teachers and speech therapists. Did their careers make them more vulnerable, or are they the type of personality which likes to solve a puzzle with group support?

There also was a majority of fair complexion and red-haired individuals. Curious. When I, a brunette, walked in the meeting, I became the second brunette in the group.

Do we have an answer why this happens? No. However there are empirical hunches. These include:

Is there a pre-disposition which gets triggered? Is there a genetic component?

Does a chemical response get miscoded? Is there an inflammatory response which does not turn off?

These are all questions that research will hopefully answer. In the meantime, remember that instead of a duck we are beautiful swans. SAR

WE ARE COMPLEX; DIAGNOSIS TAKES TIME

You are not an eggshell white, matte-finished, painted wall. Instead, you are a complex mosaic mural, different from day to day, hour to hour. You are too hot, too cold, standing, lying, hydrated or dry, calm or anxious.

All the tests, visits and studies are done to sort out these shiny tile pieces. It is a tedious process and there are numerous tests to complete.

While grasping at straws, emotional/mental labels may be bantered about. It is the outcome, not the cause? Who wouldn't be worried or anxious when vibrancy, independence and wellness has been derailed? You are a puzzle. A mystery. You are not a garden variety simple case with a direct solution or fix.

Specialty referrals abound and eventually you have an "aha" moment. No wonder, the puzzle pieces add up. The mosaic fits. There you have it _ clarity. You make sense. The light goes on and the specialist declares "we have some answers."

Take heart, diagnosis is a long process; on average it takes three to five years. SAR

PREPARING FOR DOCTOR APPOINTMENT

Appointment day has finally arrived and there are expectations to identify and treat the disorder. Be aware that health care providers do not have endless time to spend with each patient. Oftentimes, a 15–60-minute slot is allotted. When you meet the medical person, do not begin by performing an "organ recital," talking of every single complaint you experience. Rather, be organized. I lie down on the paper-covered bench in the room. This keeps brain fog at bay so that I can stay focused for the appointment. Have an outline for every visit. I suggest this format used by nurses for charting. It is called the SOAP method.

- S- subjective. These are my worries or concerns.
- S- symptoms. How often, how severe and what did I do to relieve it and did it work?
- O- objective. Bring such items as your blood pressure journal, headache diary, labs and tests done by other specialists.
- A- assessment. What do you think this is?
- P- plan. Develop a well plan which includes medications, refills and modifications. Receive letters for work and gym stating what you can do and testing referrals to specialists. Secure a follow-up appointment.

An illness plan includes how do I reach you; what symptoms warrant an emergency department visit; do my medications get modified and what over-the- counter medications can I take for a cold, headache...? With preparation, a medical appointment can be more productive for both the patient and doctor. SAR

PERSEVERE DESPITE MEDICAL TESTS, PROCEDURES

Never forget that you are the essential member of your all-star medical team.

I have had plenty of emesis basins and too many gowns that don't tie in the back. I could make a Christmas wreath with all the allergy, fall risk and identification armbands worn. I drank gallons of barium. Don't let them fool you, flavoring does not help, it all tastes nasty. I had enough blood drawn to know a competent phlebotomist from a rookie. I have had a spinal tap. My dear Ed, husband of six weeks, held me for it while I curled up.

I had five progressively worsening tilt table tests. I always hated amusement parks. Electromyography (EMG) is hideous. I despise them.

When readying for a colonoscopy, why don't doctors be honest and call them "colon explosions?" Cleanse just doesn't convey the truth.

My early referrals included specialists in hypertension, endocrine, speech and physical therapy, neuro-ophthalmology, surgery, memory, psychology, gastroenterology, and turnips. I have been x-rayed, analyzed, measured, scoped, stretched and prodded. Therefore, I chose to be grateful and advance beyond the discovery phase. It is a difficult process; made stronger by the knowledge we are seeking a strong medical team and treatment plan. SAR.

* **Definitions taken from Dysautonomia International website subcategory: Learn More What is dysautonomia; Basics of the Autonomic Nervous System; POTS; Other forms of Dysautonomia; Underlying causes of dysautonomia. www.dysautonomiainternatinal.org**

*Autonomic testing information taken from uhhopsitals.com. Patient guide to prepare for autonomic testing – autonomic testing information.**

DIARY QUESTIONS

If you have been diagnosed with a form of dysautonomia or other chronic condition, what is it?

What symptoms do you experience?

What kind of testing have you undergone and what specialists have you seen?

How has this diagnosis changed your life and how do you deal with the challenging health issues?

How do you stay hopeful despite chronic illness?

Chapter One: Transitions

"Life isn't about finding yourself. It's about creating yourself."
—Oscar Wilde

"Things do not change; we change."
—Henry David Thoreau

"Always remember that you have within you the strength, the patience and the passion to reach for the stars to change the world."
—Harriet Tubman

When a person's autonomic nervous system malfunctions, change is inevitable. There are physical changes—exhaustion, varying blood pressure and heart rate, nausea, headaches, dizziness and more. And there are emotional changes—anger, frustration, sadness, confusion, uselessness and eventually perhaps acceptance.

A transition is defined as a change from one condition to another. Transition is rampant when learning to live with dysautonomia. Socially, we lose friends; deal with remarkable feelings of loss and oftentimes must curtail or quit activities/jobs/ that we enjoy. While not everyone must termi-

nate working, both Sharon and I retired early. I had three days between the time my sick leave was scheduled until it began, resulting in retirement nine months later. Sharon, on the other hand, had no warning. A medical crisis sent her life spiraling. Read on for that life event.

LAST DAY BRINGS BIRTHS, CONFUSION, DREAD

I had an extended recovery time after four abdominal surgeries in 12 months. There was resolve to discover the cause of my persistent abdominal pain and weight loss; as I had a family history. My paternal grandmother was diagnosed with colon cancer at the age of 45. Doctors checked me for gastroparesis with an awful test using irradiated powdered eggs.

I belonged to the barium flavor-of-the-month club. I drank it by the gallon for a year. A first colonoscopy was clear. Subsequently, a second barium study showed a web of adhesions compressing the small intestines. The web was lysed, and an appendectomy revealed a chronically inflamed appendix per pathology findings.

Pain and weight loss persisted. I lost about 10 pounds monthly. A work pager, clipped to my waistband, was painful on contact. I had a laparoscopic cholecystectomy several months later and returned to work on an abbreviated schedule. These surgeries took a hit on my accrued sick time hours. The pathology report said chronic inflammation, gall bladder. Food would not get in and stay down. I consumed mostly carbohydrates and Ensure. My surgeon speculated that I had an eating disorder. This was a huge affront to me. My specialty was women's health. I had studied and was alert to signs of eating disorders, binging, and anorexia in female clients. I had been very direct with the doctor about symptoms, and my presentation did not fit a psychosocial locus. My blood pressure was never taken on post-operative checkups, despite expressing a concern about profound fatigue.

Another colonoscopy? Sure, why not. Another bowel preparation, and again huge fluid loss? The result was negative. Each of these procedures came with anesthesia. During this long recovery, I tried diligently to improve strength with exercise, good sleep, and healthy eating habits. It was my gynecologist, on a routine annual exam, who discovered that blood pressure was off kilter.

My primary care physician prescribed a blood pressure medication. I remember one day I was attending a funeral Mass and did not feel right. I looked down and my arms were cold and completely blue. My head felt like a marshmallow. I was faint, so I abruptly left the service. I thought, "not here, not now. Shoot. Better leave before they toss me in a coffin too."

Soon I was back to full schedule in the faculty practice midwifery unit. A full- time midwife worked three eight-plus hour days in clinic seeing women for gynecology or childbearing issues. My schedule was: Monday, Tuesday, Thursday, a 24-hour Friday call, and rotating weekends with colleagues.

This is my last day of working:

- On 10-21-01: 0445 alarm sounds. Jump out of bed, start a load of wash. Make coffee, shower, shampoo, dress, coffee sip and eat bagel. Unload dishwasher; transfer wet clothes to dryer. Brush teeth.
- 0610: leave home with three cans of Ensure and a grapefruit. Drop off youngest daughter at high school.
- 0640: drive to the hospital, park in garage, walk briskly to building, go to call room, change into scrubs, do hand scrub to start shift.
- 0655: get report from off-going nurse midwife. Meet student nurse midwife here for clinical practicum.
- 0700: shift begins, here I go.

I wrote the date 10-21-01 all day long. I managed six laboring women and attended each of their births. All our newborns were healthy arrivals. A birth is multifactorial: observation of labor changes over time, charting, encouragement, teaching, silent presence. Labor is difficult, physical work. We write notations, birth certificates and orders. We interface with the nursing staff and residency chief to provide progress updates.

Then came postpartum rounds on our clients who had birthed in the preceding 48 hours, in between labor checks. Rounds include physical exam, support, teaching, writing and prescriptions. We then sweep by the nursery to check on the babies and write orders for the mother's recovery needs.

I managed our patients in the triage room; a ward with six beds This included screening evaluations, ranging from sexually transmitted infection detection, false labor evaluations, trauma, or evaluation of any female greater than 20 weeks' gestation received from the emergency department. I handled all calls coming into the service phone line from clinic patients. Sleep in these 24 hours was nonexistent.

Serving as a clinical preceptor for a student nurse midwife requires ever-presence because the student works on the premise of your state licensure. It is a scrutiny of knowledge, skill, mastery of material, and behavioral technique of labor guidance. You hone skills of knowledge, manual abilities, precision and dexterity. Supervising a student on a 24-hour call is mentally challenging but rewarding. It is invigorating to see the practice through a newbie's eyes. They ask the best questions. We were awake and working hard for 24 continuous hours.

We had another admission near report off time; I was running on fumes. I gave the student a verbal progress report.

- 0700 sigh. My replacement is here and given report. Do another hand scrub, peel off scrubs, dress, and run to parking garage.
- 0710 dash home, through rush hour traffic, swoop daughter Lindsey up and cover her with kisses, because it is her birthday, and rush to get her to school. I had an enormous call, never slept, but had the silent joy of attending the birth of six babies, on

my daughter's own birthday, in the very same hospital. Each time I handed a newborn to its mother's awaiting arms, I would say: "great job; you're now a mom forever." Got Lindsey to school, and we planned to celebrate her big day at dinnertime.

- 0820 back home. Shower. Night night, take nap.
- 1410 awakened to my alarm to pick her up from school.

From this point on I have no memory, except that it is her birthday, and I love each of my daughters very much. It was a birthday I was not home to celebrate, yet I was with those six moms for their births.

I awoke a day later clueless of my whereabouts. I was in a small room, walled with curtains. I had wires everywhere, and intravenous fluids running. "Where am I? I don't even have my clothes on. What has happened to them? Where are my shoes!" Sound was huge: beeping and alarms.

I witnessed the person across from me: alarms went off, staff came running, resuscitation unsuccessful; crying, family gathered, pulled sheet. Wow. I knew what a code looked like from working emergency departments, and adult and pediatric intensive care units.

No way, what am I doing here? Then the person in the next bay: same thing. Holy smokes. No. That person coded and died. Again, crying family, covered sheet. The man in the bay next to me was talking loudly on the phone to his brother. The caller wanted to talk about the Cleveland

Browns' football game, but the patient just wanted to say he loved his brother.

The staff was obviously busy. I thought with God about how I would escape. I've got to get out of here. I had to figure out what I could give God, to bargain, to get out. Right, like that's going to happen... God has everything. There is nothing I could give Him, which He doesn't already have. "I know... I will promise never to complain again, if You let me go home."

My nurse came in. "My shoes?"

He: Oh, you are not going anywhere right now. You are in bigeminy, a dysrhythmia.

Me: "I'm scared."

He: I know you are.

Me: "No! Really scared."

He: I know, we will take this slow, day by day, and if that is not good enough, we will get through this hour by hour.

I went home several days later. I do not complain. It is liberating.

That admission swept me off my feet. I was unable to walk with my chicken legs. They were swaddled in ankle foot orthotics (AFO); I had drop foot bilaterally and I acquired a wheeled walker to prevent falls. Speech was minimal. I had trouble with phonation and word selection. Sound selection and formation was very difficult.

My rehabilitation consisted of months of physical therapy in both a gym and pool. I made progress in three increments: from use of my AFO and walker; to braces and a cane, and now just my braces. It was great to have the wheeled walker with a basket because I could sit down when tired and put belongings in the seat basket.

I had speech homework. My daughters used a flashcard method. Each level of difficulty had a different color to indicate easy, medium, and most difficult phrases. The cards went on a circular ring. If I was having a more difficult day, my kids would scale back, and have me copy their sounds. Fatigue has a strong influence on speech clarity.

I worked diligently to regain strength, stamina, and speech.

I did attempt to go back to work but was no longer well enough to maintain a position as a nurse midwife. I attempted light duty with guidance from human resources: chart reviews, and then attempted working in the pediatric call center. When my three-month probation ended, I was asked to attend a meeting with staff members, the manager and director. We gathered around a table with me as the topic. I believe they needed bench strength to tell a dual-master-degreed nurse midwife, a nurse with 30 years' experience, that she had seen better days. They sequentially told me how I did not measure up, and it was my last day. I was outnumbered. I quietly listened thinking, "I hope this never happens to you." My only comment was to the pediatrician, "may I call you if I have any further questions?" They offered to let me stay for the rest of the day shift.

"No thank you. I won't stay where I am not wanted." I left the office space, went into the hospital lobby and stretched out on a couch with my new leg braces. I waited until my kids were done with school and picked me up. I could not drive.

It would have been immeasurable sorrow to know ahead of time that 10-21-01, my last day/night 24 call, was my last day of work as a midwife. I think it was a blessing having not known. I believe that having my last day of birth attendance as a midwife, the same day as my last child's birth date, was a healing blessing.

Tough, sorrowful, surrender yes. Defeated, no. SAR

Laura's transition from work to retiring, at age 47, took a bit longer than Sharon's. Read on to discover how her career ended.

LABOR DAY: HOPING I CAN CONTINUE WORK

On Labor Day we recognize those in the work force. It's ironic as tomorrow starts another school year, and it may be my last. Dysautonomia symptoms are wreaking havoc on my body and I am unsure whether I will be able to continue in the profession as an elementary school counselor. Staff development was last week and proved challenging. In fact, after three days of work I was wiped out; I could not drive myself home; and came too close to passing out in the faculty room. Thankfully I knew to get myself on the ground and elevate feet. I stayed on the floor until I became steady enough to walk to the nurse's office with the help of a teacher friend. I spent most of the afternoon lying flat on a cot. I did perform a few duties, but mostly rested; trying to combat the feelings of nausea, headaches, light headedness, exhaustion and weakness that would not subside. I was not stable and knew I couldn't work, let alone drive.

My blood pressure continues to be orthostatic, heart rate jumps when I stand, and I easily tire. I get nauseous and have headaches. I can't stand or sit too long without symptoms and am still undergoing evaluation by a neurologist. Hopefully he will connect more pieces of this medical puzzle. While I am taking various prescriptions and vitamins, I am not better and deal with daily symptoms. I don't have days that I feel well, rather I might have an hour or two before symptoms escalate. I'm unsure how this unpredictable health will affect employment, which consists of working with elementary school-aged children 20 hours per week in addition to teachers, parents and administrators. I also work at night in our family counseling setting when necessary.

I have an appointment with my primary care physician next week in which we will discuss whether he should put me on a disability medical leave. This is not what I want to have occur but have realized it may be the only answer until the doctors can devise a solid treatment plan. Some days it takes every ounce of energy just to shower and get dressed; I can't imagine going to work on those days. I can't consistently sit upright and follow a conversation for extended amounts of time, so counseling would be difficult. I have realized that until treatment can be fine-tuned, working may be impossible.

I have had a productive career, spending 23 years as a counselor and four years as a reporter/editor of a weekly newspaper, and hopefully I will continue. If not, however, I know I have helped many children and families, and enjoyed myself in the process. This disorder is not of my choosing, and I am doing everything in my power to get better. I hope the doctors I have enlisted will do everything in their power to find the proper treatments to help me regain health.

SICK LEAVE A DIFFICULT PILL TO SWALLOW

I am exhausted, both physically and emotionally. But I can't sleep. I'm too wired as what I faced today was huge and what is to come in the next two days is even greater. It's almost midnight and I'm awake.

Today was a pivotal day. I saw Dr. David Deberny, primary care physician, and admitted what I have known for a long time - dysautonomia symptoms are not under control. It is too difficult at the present time to work. I expend much too much energy just driving three miles to school and once there I have to lie down several times during the day to prevent myself from throwing up or worse yet, passing out. That would not be a good scene considering I am an elementary school counselor working with five- to 11-year-olds.

Today when I met with the doctor and he asked how work was going, I told him what a struggle it was to even shower, let alone work. Some days it feels like I have used up all of the energy reserves before I even start the car. It is horrible.

My doctor was compassionate and knows how I have

struggled for about a year. He often sees me lying flat when he walks into the examining room, as the drive to his office usually sends my blood pressure and heart rate up, produces a headache and makes me nauseous. Lying flat stabilizes me somewhat.

Dr. Deberny remembers the old me that was full of energy and easily walked two to three miles a day but can now barely make it down the hall at school without having to rest. He knows this medical situation has been a huge struggle and seems genuinely concerned and willing to keep working to help me heal. He reassured me today that I should not feel any guilt about beginning a sick leave; that it may take a year or two to heal; and that he hopes things will indeed improve. He also reassured me that we will continue to try different treatment modalities in hopes of results. Dr. Deberny explained it as if my body is running a marathon at times and needs time to recover. While we can perform blood tests and look at some factors, we can't view all the internal workings of the body to see how the vitamins and drug regimens affect me. I am fortunate to have a doctor that works with me and shows compassion and empathy towards these struggles.

I'm not sure why I was surprised, but when I told my husband, boss, family and a few friends of the impending leave of absence, emotions erupted. I was amazed at how sad I felt. The sadness overcame me quickly; some of it I'm sure was from the genuine concern and sadness from the people I told. At 47 years old, I never expected my career may be over and that is a difficult concept to grasp. I love my career; I love where I work and the children. I don't want to leave and certainly don't want to exit on these terms. I am aware the next two days will be very difficult. Tying up loose ends, saying goodbye to children and adults and physically packing up belongings will stretch every fiber of me and I don't know how I will accomplish all that needs to be done. I just take it one moment at a time, like I have learned to do, and try to pace myself. But this is a mountain I am climbing up and over, and a grieving process I will begin. I dread it all.

LAST DAY OF WORK DIFFICULT AND HEARTBREAKING

I walked out of work today for what may be the last time, leaving behind a career as an elementary school counselor that spanned nearly 23 years. And the choice was not mine, but rather forced upon me by a body that is working improperly.

Just three days ago I finally faced the reality that I can't pretend that I am able to work. It has become more difficult to just get up, shower, dress and drive to school. And then dysautonomia produces so many crazy symptoms _ rise and drop in blood pressure and heartrate; nausea; diarrhea; hot and cold body temperatures; chills; brain fog; dizziness; presyncope; headaches; which force me to stop what I am doing and lie flat. I drink a tremendous number of fluids, eat small meals, move around a lot and take vitamins and medications. These treatments have not worked to heal me and I'm not physically strong enough to work. I am currently on an indefinite sick leave; what is believed to be at least six months but in reality, could be the first step towards permanent disability retirement.

It was surreal to walk out of school today, leaving a profession that I love. I am still good at counseling. I never wanted to leave my job like this. I planned to work for 30 years, retire and move on. Instead, I may have to retire with a much-reduced disability pension at a far-too young age. It was a big blow emotionally, even though I knew I had no other choice. I tried my best and did not fail, rather I realized my limitations, voiced them to the doctor who heard and helped me. Hopefully this will be a step closer to regaining some health and reinventing myself, with or without a profession.

LOOKING FOR ROUTINE, PEACE AT HOME

Today was a long day. It was the first of a medical leave from work. I began my leave after realizing last week that I can no longer drag myself to work. My doctor decided a mere six days ago that a sick leave is the answer. I hope that with proper medications, vitamins, rest, exercise and nutrition I will begin to live a more normal existence. God, I hope so.

What I want to do is get on my 21-speed hybrid road bike and pedal as hard as possible for miles on end to decrease some of this pent-up energy and anger I feel. Under the anger is sadness from this great loss of the life I knew before my autonomic nervous system began to break down and then went totally haywire. Pre-disorder, I would ride hills, difficult hills, until my legs would feel like mush, heart pounding and I would feel relief. Now my legs feel like mush and the heart can pound just from getting out of bed in the morning; climbing stairs; showering; doing wash or other activities. After putting the dishes away and finishing preparing dinner, I must now lie down and rest. This is not the exhilarating tired I once felt on bike rides, rather it is the annoying exhaustion of dysautonomia.

I don't want to be home during the day, I want to be working with the children whom I love. I want to see friends and interact with them and even see the parents and teachers who would sometimes annoy me. I am stuck at home and don't know what the future holds. It is unclear whether I will have to seek a disability retirement or if this rest will heal my body enough to reduce the incidences of brain fog and other symptoms. I don't want to know all that life has in store, but I sure would like to know if I am going to return to my career or if Sept. 15, 2011, was the last day of my professional school counseling career. It was a blast the 23 years I had, but I'm not ready to give it up. I know; however, it may be over.

The unknown is one of the most difficult aspects of this disorder. That and the fact it is such a trial-and-error condition. There is no exact treatment plan, rather try this and then if that doesn't work try that. See this neurologist, this endocrinologist, this cardiologist, have this blood work done, then this and so on. It is many, many medical visits and not a direct route to the solution. There are too few answers.

PRIMARY DOCTOR ASKS IF I AM DEPRESSED

I went to the doctor yesterday, four weeks after he decided I needed to begin a sick leave from work. I was impressed with him, as he mentioned it is very common to become depressed while dealing with chronic illness.

I think the most pressing question I had was about recovery. Did he think I would recover and ever return to work? The answer could cause depression.

Dr. David Deberny, who is my age, is a kind, caring man who admits he has only treated a handful of dysautonomia patients in his career. While he is confident in his treatment, he is pleased that I seek assistance from a neurologist who has an expertise in the field. Unfortunately, that neurologist, who works in another state, is moving across country. I hope the hospital replaces him and I can continue to travel the 400-mile round trip to manage treatment. In the meantime, I see my primary care doctor every one to two months.

When I asked Dr. Deberny what he thought of the probability of going back to work he said I would definitely be off at least six months and perhaps I would be unable to return and would need to seek permanent disability. Even though I knew the answer before he spoke, it was a big blow. At age 47, with three children ranging in age from eight to 16, the last thing I want is to be unemployable. I have a master's degree, worked 27 years in two professions and I'm not ready to give that up. On the other hand, my body doesn't work properly; I tire quickly; my brain fogs out and sometimes I have to stop whatever is happening immediately and urgently and lie flat so that I don't pass out. I am trying to grasp my doctor's words.

I have worked very hard to keep myself from becoming depressed. Today I peddled on and off for 20 minutes on an exercise bike. I always listen to favorite music while exercising which helps with motivation. I try to stay tuned in to our children's needs. I read with them, hug my little guy, play and talk. I even played a little soccer outside this weekend, and while it was only for about five minutes in the driveway, we all had fun.

I have a counselor I speak with when necessary. I found her when I first realized that my body was failing me, as I knew this was not going to be an easy fix and I was going to be challenged both physically and psychologically. I know I can't do this alone and I need to be challenged to keep my psyche in check. The counselor helps me to realize that while I am dealing with tremendously difficult challenges, I still have much strength and can find joy in life. I joined a Bible study group online that has enriched me spiritually. It is geared towards people with chronic illnesses.

I would not choose to have dysautonomia, but it has made me keenly aware of what is most important in life; family, friends, faith and health. I wouldn't say I am accustomed to this new reality but I'm working to stay emotionally healthy. I am fortunate my doctor has the courage to address such issues.

DELETING EMAILS BIG STEP IN CLOSING OUT CAREER

I cleared out my work e-mail today. I threw out everything. The account is blank. Why I was keeping emails is a mystery but today I decided it was time to let go.

I will receive more e-mails but most I will not read, unless I know they are directed at me, rather than a general staff e-mail. I don't need to read general e-mails as I am on a leave of absence from work and don't need to know what is happening.

I read e-mails religiously at first. I wanted to know exactly what was occurring at school. I wanted to know what meetings were held, from staff breakfasts to even curriculum meetings; something in which I don't even partake. Now I don't care about these. Some of the e-mails I don't even understand; there is new training and acronyms that I am not privy to.

Reality is sinking in and I'm beginning to believe that there is a good chance I won't work again. My stamina is low, blood pressure labile, symptoms persist, and I can't seem to go more than one or two hours without symptoms. I'm hoping I can establish a new normal that allows me a quality of life to participate in activities without having to think almost constantly about how to avoid the fogging out mentally and syncope feelings that often occur. I'd like to be able to drive longer than 20 minutes; sit at my daughter's entire basketball game; attend church; go out to lunch; shop for a bit; sit with my husband and talk at a coffee shop; go for a walk or see a movie. Working, however, may just be out of the question. I don't think I'm going to need my work e-mail account too much longer and I'm beginning to let go.

SAYING GOODBYE TO COLLEAGUES HEARTBREAKING

I am angry, sad and frustrated. It is one of the worse days of this medical journey. I feel like I have lost a huge part of my identify. I have been forced to give up something I have loved, and I have no choice in the matter.

Yesterday I took a big step; I sent an email to the staff at my elementary school letting them know that I am retiring as of July 1. I will not work again. This is not a choice and if feels like a death. My doctor and I talked about it two weeks ago and agreed my body is not operating the way it needs to for work. And if I do improve, or when I do improve the goal is for me to resume some things in my life but working is not an option.

I thought about it and decided it was time to let friends and colleagues know what was occurring. My boss knew and a few close friends, but I thought it was time to let the entire staff in on my situation. The responses I have gotten are amazing and kind. But my response for some reason surprises me. I am so sad and frustrated. I am grieving the loss of a career. It is what I loved. I didn't bring the job home much, but it was a big part of life and now it is gone. I still must go in and say goodbye to the kids and pack up a few things. To know I will never counsel at the school again is difficult. To realize my body has betrayed me is hard to understand. I'm angry, but surprised that anger has resurfaced.

I had a great career and have performed many productive things thus far in life. I enjoyed it all and have no regrets. I just wish I had more time to work with the children and families. I don't, however, and somehow, I will become settled with this in time. I know the grief process and realize I must go through it. My training tells me this. I must do what I can to deal with the grief. It will be difficult, and writing brings some solace.

I will continue to move forward and deal with the many complex feelings of this disorder.

E-MAIL SENT TO COLLEAGUES EXPLAINS RETIREMENT

This is the original e-mail I sent to the school staff telling them I would not return:

When I looked in my plan book, I saw The Peanuts final comic strip taped to Sept. 15, 2011 – the last day I worked at CAS. I had hoped I would work again. I read it and thought, wow, how profound. I loved Snoopy, cut the comic strip out of the newspaper in 2000 and kept it all those years. In this final comic strip Snoopy is sitting on his doghouse thinking with a typewriter in front of him. The message, by Charles Schultz, thanks the reader for 50 years of enjoyment. He goes on to say he is unable to continue with this schedule. He expresses gratefulness for the love and support of fans.

That last day of work I put this comic in my plan book, wrote last day and closed the book. Yesterday when I read it I thought hmmm interesting. I started out as a reporter in 1985, my first career, loved writing and still do. In

1989 I began my elementary school counseling career. I'm not sure how 23 years have gone by, but I am thankful for them.

It is time to tell you that I am retiring from my job as an elementary school counselor. I was going to ask Trena (the school principal) to tell you at a staff meeting but that isn't fair to her. I found this cartoon and it seems to share my sentiments. I had a tremendous ride and have loved it all, both careers.

I am settled with the idea of retiring; have a good support system and am enjoying writing about this crazy medical journey that continues. I was in Cleveland again Friday and will continue to seek treatment; eventually my autonomic nervous system might heal a bit and give me an increase in better moments.

I have learned to enjoy the little things in life that give me joy; and look back on a career with no regrets. I realize I have done some good in this world. I would prefer not to retire at the age of 47, but God doesn't always give us what we want, and it is what it is _ but I am ok with this.

I ask you to do me one thing; enjoy today. Grumble if you must as we all do. But find joy in your every day. Even in the darkest times there is joy to be had. Try to have fun each day. I try, and it makes each day better.

I will be in before the year is out to say goodbye. Peace, Laura

GRANTED: TO BESTOW OR CONFER UPON

At 2 p.m., March 8 I found the courage to call the New York State Teacher's Retirement System to ask the outcome of the medical board's review of my application for a disability pension. Every fiber in me wanted to continue in the profession. However, my body revolted against that idea and my doctor kindly helped me come to the realization that I could not work.

At 47, I never dreamt I'd retire. So when I heard the word "granted" it was bittersweet to put it mildly.

I hung up and called my husband. His response was so kind I cried. I sat in silence for some time in disbelief, sadness and relief. This part was over; my retirement system believed me and it was a relatively easy process. One down, one to go (social security _ that had already been a much more difficult process in just the amount of paperwork that had to be filed).

THE WAKE- RECOGNIZING THE END OF A CAREER

Nothing in life prepared me for the loss of my career. I returned to graduate school midlife and had just made my final student loan payment.

When I became sick, I had a very slow recovery from four abdominal surgeries in two years. I made numerous attempts to work, with the help of my director, human resources department, and colleagues. I performed light duty, short days, every other half-day and other combinations to improve stamina. I even transferred to two different departments to 'test drive' the workload. There were numerous 'good-byes.'

Leaving a career is a huge loss. You lose your title, rank, friends, acquaintances, salary, routine and connected networking. You let go and release so much of what you thought defined you. Physical limitations are insurmountable, and you assess what is left of your identity and life.

The process is like a set of LEGOs; what pieces are left and what can I rebuild after the crash?

I was aware of how much physical therapy, speech therapy, strength and endurance work I did faithfully to regain stamina. I had numerous specialist consultations and medications. Many nights I would take off walking around my block, get weak, pause and lean by the mailboxes along the route.

When the reality finally settled in, I became very angry. I took boxes and tossed professional textbooks inside. With help from my future husband, we lugged about four packed boxes into the basement and stuffed them on the shelf in a closet. Then I sobbed. I truly thought my heart was broken. My fiancé held me until the crying stopped. That was the wake. I had to grieve by action the permanent loss.

What's left? My spirit; the divine light within me. I belong to a very small exclusive club of those who appreciate tiny things: walking, talking, having good veins, being sent home after a squad trip to the emergency room or hospital. We pull over for ambulances because we have ridden in them and understand the urgency. We reach a level of gratitude few ever attain. There is a highly developed sense of humor. Who worries about shaved legs with a labile blood pressure?

What is important to me? I choose to celebrate good things, not worry about the small things. SAR

NEW SCHOOL YEAR MAKES HOUSE TOO QUIET

The house is quiet, my family is back at school, and I am home with the music blasting to hide the too-still home. This is the first year in 41 that I am not going to school; either as a student (in my formative years, college and graduate school) or counselor. I officially retired July 1, 2012, or as I put it retirement chose me when dysautonomia stole my career.

I barely worked the first three weeks of the 2011-12 school year and then went out on a medical leave of absence that eventually led to retirement. Today begins the school year for everyone except me. During the hustle and bustle of getting the family ready _ one fourth grader, one ninth grader, one 12th grader and one school principal _ I went about my business taking pictures of each after ingesting 26 pills to get the day started. I drank 32 ounces of Gatorade, did physical therapy exercises to help reduce pain from recent shoulder surgery and hoped my stomach would cooperate so I would be able to stand at the bus stop with the youngest while he waited for his ride (it did). Heck, my legs even cooperated today as did the rest of me. We were outside just long enough for a few pictures before the bus stopped.

I am left listening to music wondering how I am going to fill the day. I know I will exercise soon but after that I have no idea. It is not a matter of what I do today but the future. I am doing alright emotionally but worry and hope that today does not set me back in the grieving process. Dysautonomia robs us of a lot and I have worked to establish a new sense of self. Days like today hit me in the face and make me realize how much I have lost and how life has changed drastically.

Today I give myself permission to do whatever comes my way. Tomorrow I must get back up and start again, remembering I have come a long way and will continue to grow emotionally in this journey.

CONCERT PRODUCES JOY AND RESPITE FROM SADNESS

I dreaded the day, the year anniversary of leaving my job as an elementary school counselor. The day I walked out of school I hoped I would go back. Instead, eight months later my chronic illness forced retirement.

When the anniversary approached this fall, I thought I would have a really difficult time emotionally. A remarkable thing happened instead. I miscalculated the anniversary date by one day and missed it. Phew, it was yesterday, I thought, and I had survived. Heck, I didn't survive, actually I thrived. In retrospect I celebrated the day without even knowing it. I did something rare for me now, I went to a concert.

I saw Grammy-award winning singer Amy Grant on the spur of the moment. She played in a tiny venue of 1,200 people. With some modifications I loved the show. I found balcony seats on the aisle and when I became symptomatic my husband and I went out into the corridor to stretch. Much to my surprise we had the hallway to ourselves; acoustics were wonderful, and it was as if we had our own private concert hall. It felt like paradise.

We ate salted popcorn and I hung out enjoying the music; our first date in many months. It was a glorious time to be out experiencing life. The following day I crashed; exhausted and feeling all the symptoms of this disorder. But I did not care one bit. I had a great time, and it was well worth it, and that is what is most important. I am choosing to live, to experience, to have fun and it is worth the pain and exhaustion that follows. Sure, would I like to feel normal and not have to sacrifice for a good time? Of course. Will I do it again? Absolutely. Will I crash again? Sure, but I will be ok with this. Because it was a memory, it is life, and I am choosing to live the best I can.

TAKING LIFE INVENTORY A YEAR AFTER RETIRING

I've been officially retired for a year. I've said that retirement chose me, rather than the other way around, as having a chronic illness forced the issue.

It was an eventful year with ups and downs, both emotionally and physically. Today I realized, while seeing a former colleague at Starbucks, that I have settled in to retirement. We talked about the kids and the joy it is to work with them, but she reminded me of the drudgery that sometimes comes with other aspects of the job. I wished her well and told her what a real blessing it was talking with her; she said she needed to hear that affirmation.

This got me thinking that there are some real perks of retirement; even if I am not close to the "official" retirement age, most of the hairs on my head are red, rather than grey and I would work if I was able.

I wanted to share a few of these perks with you:

I don't have to wear dress clothes and panty hose each day, although I do have a collection of compression stockings that rival most older people.

If I want to have a chocolate chip cookie for breakfast I do with a Starbucks iced tea. You see, if I have the energy to get to Starbucks I can indulge. My weight, while not perfect, does not fluctuate much since being diagnosed. My appetite is poor. Sometimes I must remember to eat and oftentimes protein shakes are easiest. If I can eat, great, no one is going to judge me for having an occasional treat.

I don't have to attend events I don't find pleasurable or are too lengthy or difficult to get to. I don't have the energy.

I relish the relationships I have. It takes great effort to stay upright at times, so if I am talking to someone and visiting, I find myself very present in the conversation.

LABOR DAY NOT AS DIFFICULT AS ANTICIPATED

My daughter started her junior year of high school today; my husband opened a new school; my youngest began sixth grade and oldest went back to college.

The school year is filled with possibilities, challenges, opportunities and unknowns.

It is also a reminder that I no longer am employed. This begins my third year of retirement and I sit at Starbucks sipping iced tea, listening to music and writing. Tea, writing and music are three things I enjoy. It is only 8:30 a.m. but after dropping my daughter at school I could choose to go home and do laundry or head to Starbucks and write. I chose the latter.

My body is stronger/healthier than it was three years ago. Today I even had that fleeting thought while dressing that perhaps I could work again. But my body is unpredictable. I didn't think I was going to make it out of a store in an upright position recently. The aftereffects included a stomach that exploded at a nearby store; a lasting headache and exhaustion.

I am enjoying life more but also seem to be crashing a bit more. It is a trade-off that I'm willing to risk if I don't put myself in danger.

September always brings reminders of the great loss of my career. I never planned to retire early. When I left school on September 15, 2011, for the last time I had hoped I would come back from an extended sick leave. Deep down I knew my body was betraying me as if I was on a horrible roller coaster ride that had no beginning or end. Thankfully the roller coaster slows down some now and occasionally stops so I can breathe. Unfortunately, though, it starts up again, sometimes slowly other times very quickly; either way producing ugly results.

Although my career ended abruptly, I had a blast doing the job and for that I am thankful. As I have told many people a career is important, but we also need to enjoy the other aspects of our lives. While I still feel the sting of a lost career, I need to remember my words and embrace this detour.

Labor Day - a reminder of so much. Perhaps someday it will be a happier holiday.

MEMORIES OF LAST WORK DAY STILL VIVID

It has been three years since I walked out of the elementary school in which I worked. I can remember many moments of that last day of work. These include driving to work listening to my favorite band the Goo Goo Dolls sing "Feel the Silence;" counseling the last two boys; carting boxes to the car with fifth grade helpers; and asking God what he was doing in front of a dear friend, the school nurse, as we both fought tears and lost. I remember finally hanging up keys in the office, walking down that quiet hall one last time and exiting the school with a colleague who carried my gift plant.

What a day it was, knowing I was leaving a career on sick leave but realizing in my heart that time was up. My body was not going to miraculously recover and allow a return to work. I tried each day to drag myself to school. I wasn't successful and there were many times when I was left lying flat either in the nurse's office or mine trying to stabilize a revolting body. I came too close to passing out too many times and while I loved the job I was exhausted. Each day I had fantasies of lying down on the bench in the front foyer and sleeping - for hours.

Yea, it was not working. So I left. And it was horrible.

And I still mourn. Especially in September when everyone else goes back to school and I don't. I hate it. But my head knows I can't work. Every few months, however, I say to my husband or doctor "do you think I could work?" The answer is always the same - and I know it - but when I have a string of good moments thoughts get carried away.

But they are moments not hours.

And I am trying to be thankful for them.

And three years ago, I could not do all the things I can now.

Five years ago I could do so much more. That thought produces frustration and sadness; especially when I think about all the effort it takes to sit in a chair, stand, attend to things and just live.

Sometimes the anger is great, the sadness overwhelming. I wish I could have a healthy body. I tire of persevering, managing symptoms, pretending I am ok when I am not. But if I don't fight to manage the symptoms my body will spiral downward. I do what I need to do and remember that I am blessed. Regardless of the trials, I am alive, living the best I can with the people I love. And for that I am grateful.

TIPS FOR FILING APPLICATION FOR SOCIAL SECURITY

I was surprised at how thorough the social security disability insurance application process is. I applied online, without legal help, and was approved on the first attempt. Most people told me to hire a lawyer, but I didn't. I will tell you why. If you are not a spiritual person just skip over my explanation in the next paragraph.

On Oct. 4, 2011, my oldest son made his Confirmation, which is a big ceremony in our church. I was excited and all I wanted was to be able to see him receive this sacrament. The mass was three-hours long and the church packed. I had to leave several times and went in the chapel; a favorite place, to stretch. My husband texted me so I didn't miss my son's Confirmation. The event was purely joyful, and I felt the Holy Spirit in that church. I had to leave soon after and went outside to get Gatorade from the car. When I came back into the chapel, I became very symptomatic; the cold weather had gotten a hold of me. My limbs were heavy and all I could do was lie on a bench and pray. I thought I was going down, and thought great, they are going to carry me out of here on a stretcher. I was freezing, foggy and stuck. I knew if I could get back in the church, I would warm up but couldn't move. I prayed. And then a voice said to me "everything will be ok even if you can't work." I had just begun a sick leave from work, but I was not thinking about that when this occurred. I was tremendously vulnerable at this point. Eventually I recovered, returned to church and slowly came out of the fog. It was some night. That message helped me to experience a total peace about the SSDI process. I won't forget that experience and often remember "everything will be okay even if you can't work."

Here are some suggestions for applying for SSDI.

PREP WORK NEEDED BEFORE APPLYING FOR BENEFITS

Secure the names of all the doctors you have seen, dates, and what tests they ordered. I went back two years and put down every doctor, even the ones that did not help me, diagnose me or have anything to do with dysautonomia. They are still part of the medical file.

Fill out the spaces for medical conditions and then treatments received. I completed this section with detail. This was a paper trail of all the doctors I went to that eventually lead to a diagnosis. Make sure you have this information before starting the process. Call the primary doctor or specialist if you need help recreating this information. I pulled out a calendar and could piece together a lot of information from that. You also need to write down as many tests and dates that you remember. Here are a few I included, perhaps these will help jog your memory: TTT, blood tests, EKG, autonomic testing, ENG, sleep study, gastric testing, scope of nose, MRI, cat scan, EMG, colonoscopy, endoscope, echocardiogram with color flow of heart, breathing test, hearing test and 30-day-heart monitor test.

List all your medications, jobs, salary, if you work and if not why. I put the reason I don't work is because of my condition.

BE THOROUGH WITH REMARKS ON APPLICATION

There is a place to add remarks. Here is an abbreviated summary of what I wrote:

I have a neurological condition called dysautonomia. The impact on my ability to be an elementary school counselor is profound and permanent. My vital signs are unstable and prevent the ability to conduct both individual and group counseling sessions. For example, I am unable to sit for longer than 10 minutes at a time. I am unable to maintain a reasonable blood flow to the brain, making it impossible to be an active listener. This disorder has totally depleted my ability to concentrate, to record to gather information and to be a therapeutic member of the school's faculty...Standing also causes symptoms. I sweat, flush, swoon, slump to the floor or the nearest wall to prop up my legs to get blood flow back to the heart. I hobble to the bathroom because my GI tract, as it loses blood flow, causes massive diarrhea. My speech becomes affected, as I struggle for clarity of thought. This is incompatible with a school...I pace my steps, energy and tasks.

WHAT INFORMATION NEEDED FOR APPLICATION?

I included letters in the claim. I believe these were helpful. I mailed letters to both the address of my case worker (local) and the address in which I returned my forms. I sent a letter from my principal, stating all the accommodations she made to help me continue working; the school nurse who wrote a medical letter stating what she observed when I spent hours in her room unwell; and my primary care doctor. The doctor said I was diagnosed with autonomic dysautonomia and NCS, was unable to perform regular work obligations and was considered to be fully, permanently disabled. His letter said I was on multiple medications, received IV fluids, saw several specialists but symptoms remain severe and persistent and affect quality of life. He did not anticipate I would be able to return to work.

I also sent three years of attendance records. My attendance was consistent until I became sick, then attendance dramatically declined.

SUGGESTIONS ON WHAT TO OMIT FROM APPLICATION

The SSDI reviewers do not seem interested in emotions. Facts are important. State that you cannot perform your job. You have tried to perform; accommodations have been made but you are unsuccessful.

DAILY LIVING SURVEY IS DEPRESSING

The Social Security Administration also sends out a lengthy, depressing daily living survey. It consists of questions ranging from can you cook a meal, to can you lift things, to can you do wash to what is your typical day? I was told to answer these questions as if I was having my worse day (and when I filled it out I was). In other words, be brutally honest. For instance, I can take a shower for two minutes on a good day; one minute on a bad day and if it is horrible day can't take a shower because I am so unstable in the shower and may pass out. My husband does the grocery shopping as I can't. He makes the meals. Sometimes I can walk to the mailbox, some days I can't. If you have a good day, don't base your answers on that day, base it on all the other days, because as we know we really don't have good days we have good moments in our days. It is impossible for many of us to work.

I also wrote a letter explaining my career, what my duties entailed, how I tried to perform them and how I could not succeed due to the worsening condition. I talked about how I loved the career but could not perform it anymore because my body would not cooperate, giving brief examples.

Minor children also qualify for benefits if you receive

benefits. Once I qualified, I called the 800 number and they set up an appointment and called me at that time on the phone. I was asked a few questions, the kids qualified, and they received their first direct deposit shortly after. Children receive one-half of your benefit total until they are 18 years old or out of high school. If you get $1500, the kids will get $750 total no matter the number of children.

FINAL THOUGHTS ON APPLYING FOR DISABILITY

This process is difficult, depressing and challenging but imperative. And I understand I was fortunate to be approved without delay. The initial benefit application online is a few pages. I thought I was done and thought wow that is easy, but no, then the fun begins - the adult disability report. Do not do this form until you have all your information. This took me about 18 hours to complete and I almost sent it in without proofing it. I was very foggy at times completing it. As a writer, I looked at the application as the biggest writing job of my life.

Remember to make copies of all your forms. Always ask for case notes from your doctors after visits. Keep everything in a binder, organized. Continue to keep medical records after approval as they review the case periodically and the records are also helpful to you at times.

Once approved, the Social Security Administration will do follow-up assessments. For me this has included filling out a form stating two years of appointments and reasons for such. This is time consuming as we have a lot of appointments. Keep track of your appointments always so you can fill out these forms more efficiently.

TIPS FOR LEAVING AND/OR RETIRING FROM WORK

Leaving a job is a difficult task if unexpected. Here are some suggestions to assist with the transition.

- Forgive. Forgiveness is a gift you give yourself. There will be those who speculate that you are a slacker or malingerer. Some may label you as having a conversion disorder. You are none of these things and you did nothing wrong to receive this diagnosis.

- Work closely with human resources and your direct supervisor. Rise above the grovel. Be grateful and polite, it will dazzle them. Take notes of every conversation: date and recall topic, discussion, and plan.

- Hang on to your pay stubs and all paperwork from doctor visits.

- Journal: phrases, dates, experiences. Sometimes there are no words but try. It will be invaluable to you later. Documentation reaches clarity.

- Lastly, I learned the importance of active listening. Be still, greet the speaker's gaze, and wait. If you feel the need to do something, just nod. Powerful words, which validate are "I believe you."

RECOMMENDATIONS FOR HANDLING GRIEF/LOSS

Grief is a natural response to loss. It is the emotional suffering we feel when something or someone we love is taken way. The more significant the loss the more intense the grief.

When dealing with the loss of health, there are several factors involved. There are the tangibles _ loss of job, relationships and money. There are intangibles _ loss of energy, brain functioning and strength. Either way, grief is difficult to handle, and support is necessary. Here are some suggestions for dealing with grief and loss:

- Find support. This could include joining an online or in-person support group, seeking a counselor or talking to a confident. There are too many emotions and situations that develop to do this on our own. Support is essential.
- Remember there is no right or wrong way to grieve, as long as you are not hurting yourself or someone else in the process. Each person grieves differently.
- The grief process takes a long time to go through and there are no shortcuts. Sometimes even when dealing with the vast losses we think we are "over it" but something else reminds us of the complexities of living with chronic conditions.
- Feeling sad, lonely, angry and frightened are normal responses. Verbalize these to someone you trust.
- Find things to do to still enjoy moments. Write, read, journal, paint, draw, listen to music, pet your dog, read to your kids, go outside in the sunshine, watch a funny television show, do a craft you enjoy; anything that gives you some peace and enjoyment.
- Garner strength through your faith; pray.
- Take care of yourself the best you can. Try to get washed and dressed daily.

- Don't let others tell you how to feel. Let yourself experience whatever you feel.

- Plan ahead for grief triggers. These include anniversaries, holidays and milestones that may bring the grief to the forefront. If the grief becomes overwhelming and you find you cannot function day-to-day you may be depressed. Seek professional help.

- If you are looking for a therapist, ask for recommendations from friends or other people you trust. Verify that your insurance covers therapy and if not ask the therapist about a sliding scale if your finances are challenged. Talk to the therapist over the phone. Ask their credentials and experience with people with medical complexities and grief. Find out what their approach to therapy is and then schedule an appointment. Give the therapist a couple sessions before you decide if they may be of help to you. Realize that therapy cannot be successful unless you are honest and put work into improving your life.

DIARY QUESTIONS

What changes have you experienced as a result of your chronic condition(s)?

How do you handle such changes?

If you have had to leave a career, what have you found helpful in finding a new routine? And did you perform a ritual, like Sharon did, when you left?

Who is in your circle that provides support in helping you deal with health challenges? Is there anyone else you need to enlist?

Chapter two: Pacemaker

"Healing is a matter of time, but it is sometimes a matter of opportunity."
—Hippocrates.

"All the knowledge I possess everyone else can acquire, but my heart is all my own,"
—Johann Wolfgang Von Goethe

"I have chosen to be happy because it is good for my heart."
—Voltaire

Each person with dysautonomia will have their own medical maze to navigate. Since several body systems are effected by dysautonomia, one might see any of these doctors: neurologist, cardiologist, endocrinologist, ophthalmologist, surgeon, primary care doctor, allergist and immunologist, gynecologist, chiropractor, physical therapist, therapist, dentist and gastroenterologist.

Symptoms develop differently for each person. In my case, I began having minor heart issues in my early 20's after a bout of mononucleosis. I remember feeling a bit off - tired, heart rate slow and odd sensation while breathing. I went *through testing and was deemed to have a healthy heart. Still at times my heart rate would slow to an uncomfortable low. I often would go for a run to speed things up, then rest. Typically, the next day I felt better.*

After living this way for nearly three decades and having a heart that seemed to continuously lose beats, I was offered a pacemaker. The pacemaker is not a cure for dysautonomia; rather it provides a means for my heart to operate at a minimal rate of 62 beats per minute. The following is my experience with undergoing a pacemaker implant.

I WANT TO ESCAPE FROM THIS NEW CHALLENGE

I wish I could get in my car and drive for hours; or ride my bike up and down steep hills, to escape, where no one locates me for a while. I would think, pray, sweat, release anger and feel my heart beating hard within my chest.

But that is the problem. I can't do these things and I can't get my heart to beat consistently at a higher rate. I am angry; actually sad and frustrated. My heart has slowly lost beats for about 25 years but lately, since being diagnosed with dysautonomia more than two years ago, I've dealt with daily bradycardia. The medical definition of bradycardia is heart rate that falls below 60 beats per minute. Most days the heartbeat hovers in the mid-high 40s until I take medication that increases it to about 60 beats per minute. Even with these medications my heartbeat barely rises and almost always drops in the 40s at night when most symptomatic. Two 24-hour heart monitor tests done a year apart noted bradycardia 50 percent of the time.

Despite best efforts my heart just won't beat more quickly. I can get it up if I stand still for a few minutes. Of course, then I am light-headed, nauseous and need to dive flat as I fight presyncope; hence my POTS diagnosis. My heart rate rises to about 90 after an hour on an exercise bike. Most healthy hearts go well beyond 120 after an hour of exercise. However, mine does not come close and dips back down quickly once exercise ceases. I learned this has a medical term—chronotropic incompetence—the heart's inability to adjust the rate to changing needs.

I saw Dr. Blair Grubb, director of the clinical cardiac electrophysiology program at the University of Toledo Heart and Vascular Center, this week. It was my third visit to the center in a year and the second to him. He recommended implanting a BIOTRONIK Evia pacemaker. Funny thing was on the 300- mile drive to Toledo I knew we would discuss a pacemaker. Yet when Dr. Grubb said we could implant it now or in two years, but he recommends it now, my reaction was surprising.

I would like to ignore my slow heartbeat; the same one that keeps me from sleeping each time it drops below a certain point, as breathing becomes uncomfortable and I feel scared. I want to turn back time to the 49-year-old women with dysautonomia, autonomic neuropathy and Ehlers- Danlos Syndrome who must rest sometimes for a myriad of reasons including a slow heartbeat. I want to believe I am managing dysautonomia well and it is no big deal. I can't do that. Rather I must make a choice about when to have a pacemaker implanted. And once I do my life will again change forever, medically.

I will have a constant reminder that I have a heart that could not keep a normal beat on its own. This process both excites and frightens me.

PACEMAKER MAY PROVIDE MISSING ENERGY

In five weeks I will receive a BIOTRONIK Evia pacemaker. I received the phone call from Dr. Grubb's office today to schedule the procedure. What will take a mere one to two hours to implant has caused a lot of anxiety since I heard about the impending surgery 15 days ago. Surgery is scheduled in 35 days.

On the morning of October 9 at the University of Toledo Medical Center in Ohio, I will be fitted with the pacer. I wish the day was here so I could get it over with, yet I would like to skip surgery altogether as I am scared. It's a paradox in the greatest sense. I can choose to postpone surgery and deal with bradycardia. But that is not a great option as I feel crummy with a heart rate lower than 47.

Since discovering on Aug. 20, 2013, that Dr. Grubb thought it would be best to put in the pacemaker sooner, rather than later, a funny thing has occurred; my heart has gotten slower. I am not sure about this. I think what is happening is I am more aware of the bradycardia. I tend to minimize symptoms and just live the best I can, regardless of how badly I feel on any given day. If I exercise and then must lie down, I do that. If I shower and must rest, I do; then get back up, dressed and keep going. If I must run to the bathroom for my stomach to explode (my term for urgent diarrhea) I do then lie down, get back up and try again. Some days this can constitute the entire 24 hours, other days are better. I don't pay much attention to how slowly my heart beats The last two weeks, however, I have noticed the consistent low beats and how tired I am. Perhaps, just perhaps, this pacer will give me a bit more energy.

On Dec. 26, 2010, I woke up and could not get off the couch. I experienced my first serious case of dehydration and had the first (of many) IV hydrations. Nearly a month later, I returned to work and health spiraled out of control. I remember then, and several times since, asking my primary care doctor if there was a pill for energy. But he could never prescribe one. Dr. Grubb did prescribe Adderall, which increased blood pressure and heart rate thus giving me some energy. Unfortunately, the medication does not help sustain a steady heart rate for me. Dr. Grubb is now providing me with another opportunity for energy in the form of a pacemaker.

Here I sit, full circle. I have another chance for that elusive energy I've searched for during the last three years. It is the same energy that used to burst out of me. I still have enthusiasm and zest for life, spirit if you will, but a body that cannot keep up with what the mind wants to accomplish. Perhaps, just perhaps, this pacer will give me a fraction of that energy back. Scary, hell yes. Worth a shot, hell yes.

MAIL PRODUCES BOTH FEAR AND EXCITEMENT

The mail brought reality from the University of Toledo Medical Center in the form of preoperative instructions.

Before opening the envelope, I said to myself, ok give me a song (God) to help me through. I turned on my iPad. Out of the 305 songs on the playlist this is what I heard from Phillip Phillips;

> Hold on, to me as we go
> As we roll down this unfamiliar road
> And although this wave (wave) is stringing us along
> Just know you're not alone
> Cause I'm gonna make this place your home
> (Home by Phillip Phillips).

This song stopped me in my tracks. First, I rarely have listened to it, don't know when I uploaded it and was not aware of the lyrics. But the words are pertinent. Yes, I am going down an unfamiliar road, pacemaker surgery. I am having trouble sleeping since finding out about the surgery 21 days ago. Thoughts of a pacemaker taking over the natural, albeit slow beats of my heart, fill my mind. I am getting better at focusing on other things but am still fearful.

> Settle down, it'll all be clear
> Don't pay no mind to the demons
> They fill you with fear
> The trouble it might drag you down
> If you get lost, you can always be found
> Just know you're not alone
> Cause I'm gonna make this place your home.

Demons have haunted my dreams; I have woken in fear and sadness. I'm exhausted. and dragged down. I know I am not alone. I have a small group of trusted confidents, starting with my husband, I have chosen to tell of the surgery before it occurs. They will support me on this journey and help me remain calm as the day approaches. I have a top-notch dysautonomia specialist who predicts that a pacemaker is going to improve energy and quality of life. He has implanted more than 2,000 devices, many on people with similar symptoms of me. And of course I have faith and knowledge that God will walk this journey with me. The pacemaker will find a new "home" inside my chest; and in the process I will be reminded I am not alone in this journey dealing with dysautonomia.

BIKE RIDE PROVIDES HOPE OF BETTER LIFE

I thought about it for two weeks before finally grabbing my helmet and gloves and hopping on the bike to see how my body would perform. I hoped to go at least once around the neighborhood block - which is a mile- after being unable to ride. The weather was a perfect 70 degrees with no wind. I rationalized, with 13 days before surgery to implant a pacemaker, what could go wrong? I was willing to take the risk that I might become dizzy, need to jump off the bike and dive to the ground.

The risk was worth it.

I don't think I can adequately describe the pure joy I felt while riding. I used my brakes a little at the beginning; until I became accustomed to that amazing feeling of speed while pedaling through the neighborhood. My legs burned, despite the hours spent on the indoor recumbent bike. My heart pounded, that wonderful thump that occurs when it is being worked. It was a glorious feeling. I could not get the heartrate up to 100 bpm, but at least it came close. The blue skies, the fresh air, the sound of gears shifting as I went up and down hills; all wonderful sensory experiences I have missed for so long. It was so sweet I could nearly taste the joy.

Almost four miles in—I never expected to make it that far—symptoms of dysautonomia reared its ugly head. Who cared, I thought, and chose to push a bit further. Not the smartest move, but I made it home after traveling 4.8 miles in 30 minutes. It was a slow pace but it was a ride by someone who had not gotten on their Specialized bike in more than a year. I wanted to scream to the heavens in thanks.

As I sat drinking Gatorade looking up at the gorgeous sky, I could not help but think that just maybe this new pacemaker would allow more of these days. I could regain one of my greatest losses- biking. That would be amazing. I have to hope.

TWO DAYS BEFORE SURGERY AND FEAR INCREASES

Two days to go until a pacemaker is implanted under my collarbone.

This morning I woke up wondering whether my heart will stop, and I will die when the surgeon threads the leads.

My daughter also exhibited stress. She is 15 and cried

on the way to school, complaining of a stomachache. When she blurted out that she wanted to stay home because I was leaving tomorrow to travel five hours to the hospital where Dr. Grubb works, I knew she needed to attend school. Sure, it saddened me, but I also knew going to school would be healthier than hanging with a mom who was getting two bags of IV saline while resting on the couch. She went to school, and I pushed the thoughts of dying partially out of my head.

I know anxiety is normal. After all I was a school counselor for 23 years. I was accustomed to dealing with people's emotions, helping with life's challenges. I know all my emotions - disbelief, sadness, anger, frustration, excitement, anxiety, hopefulness - are normal. I also realize this is a life changer and may restore energy that dysautonomia stole when it slowed my heartbeat.

The seven weeks from 8/20 when Dr. Grubb said he believed it was time for a pacemaker until today have sped by quickly in one sense but slowly in another. I want the surgery over so I can get on with life, yet it is still a scary proposition which literally leaves my stomach in knots.

If I am honest with myself, I have known for about 25 years that a pacemaker was in the future. There were clues. Before I was even married, I remember going out for runs to try to increase my heartbeat because it was too slow. There were also days, many, in which I would need to go to sleep early not feeling well (bradycardia) and wake up normal the next day. There was also the moment after a surgery in which the nurse wondered if I was an athlete because my heart rate dipped so low and did not recover for a while. Sure, I always exercised but not enough for the heart rates I experienced.

Cardiac tests were performed, and all were normal. Then gradually the frequency of my heart slowing became more prominent until finally bradycardia was mentioned. In Dec. 2010 a flu bug seemed to kick dysautonomia into high gear; which eventually lead to talk of a pacemaker.

The process spanned nearly three decades and finally took a pivotal turn on 8/26/13 when I made the decision to undergo surgery. I know it is the right choice for even after taking morning medications today to increase heartbeat, I am only running at 56 beats per minute.

My bags are packed, and I am ready to travel the 300 miles each way to Toledo, Ohio for the surgery Oct. 9. My head knows it is time for the pacer and my heart continues to follow slowly behind.

POSITIVE DECISION AFFIRMED SOON AFTER SURGERY

I thought, prayed and worried for seven weeks about the decision and action I was about to undertake. And then in 90 minutes, on a sunny October day, it was over. I awoke with a pacemaker in my 49-year-old body, 300-miles from home at the University of Toledo Medical Center.

My husband was there, as was the pleasant nurse supervisor who had assured me the operation would go smoothly. I remember a little of it; moving my feet and being told to stay still; but not much more.

From the time the cardiologist suggested we do the

surgery until the actual date, I prepared. I met with my parish priest, attended a healing mass, spoke to a couple close confidents, had several sessions with my counselor, prayed, researched the pacemaker and talked to my primary care doctor. It was reassuring that internist Dr. David Deberny showed enthusiasm about the surgery. His confidence helped me move forward.

The surgery was both a frightening and exciting proposition. Frightening to think someone would insert two leads into the ventricles of my heart connected to a silver-dollar-sized machine that would help it beat. Turns out it assists my heart almost nonstop as I can't often get the resting rate to 60 beats per minute on its own. It is exciting because this little technological wonder responds to both heart rate and blood pressure, giving me an optimum chance for improved functioning.

I can't help but pause and give thanks for the medical care I have received. I have a top-notch specialist, one who people travel throughout the world to see. He is kind, smart, skilled and funny. He has given me back a huge amount of hope that life can be a bit more fulfilling as I wake up each day with a steady pulse. I have more energy and realize I am blessed to have had the opportunity for this medical care. I am literally excited to have a heart that beats steadily and allows me to do a little more before resting.

I am fortunate to have a loving family and dear friends. Chronic illness has allowed me the opportunity to savor the blessings in life. I have met new people and have had opportunities afforded me through illness. When my autonomic nervous system essentially misfired, I would never have imagined the life I have today. Sure, there have been losses but there have been many gains. Every day as I awake, I am reminded of these blessings.

It starts each day with a beautiful, steady heartbeat and gets better as the day progresses.

THREE DAYS POST-OPERATIVE AND FEELING BETTER

If I did not have a scar below my collarbone, pain and soreness, I would not know I had a pacemaker.

It is a sunny Saturday afternoon as I sit on my friend Sharon's deck listening to music and writing. My husband drove me 150 miles from University of Toledo Medical Center so I could recoup for a few days before traveling another 200 miles home. The quiet home with friends seemed like a good idea as any mother knows going back to three kids means little or no rest. Dysautonomia makes traveling difficult; add surgery to the mix and I decided taking the trek home in two phases was ideal.

What is different about life with a pacemaker? There is a scar, and it hurts; especially when I move in certain directions. I have been instructed to not lift my left arm above the shoulders as this could dislodge the two leads connected to the heart. Should this happen surgery is required. I am unsure how you know this but surmise the pacer stops pacing and pain is involved. I forgot in the shower and put my arm up while washing my hair but quickly pulled it back.

My neck and shoulders hurt. I wonder if this may be from the positioning of the body in both surgery and sleep. I sleep on my stomach and side but now must position on my back with the left arm propped on a pillow. I have slept well one of three nights.

What is amazing is I can stand a little longer without feeling symptomatic. I also took two showers without any symptoms; which has not occurred in years.

My heart no longer falls to 40-50 beats per minute, and I am unaware of it beating for the most part.

The pacer is set to begin working at 60 bpm, meaning if the heart rate falls below 60 it operates. Basically, it paces nearly nonstop. It paces up to 80 bpm at rest and to 110 for movement. These are conservative settings but after some discussion in the hospital of concerns of going too high with the rates, my doctor set these parameters.

I feel good. Granted I have not exercised yet. I have rested, eaten, showered and visited friends. So when I get home and feel ready I will get on a stationary bike and see how that feels.

Seventy-hours post-operative and things are stable. I am hopeful. That is all I can really ask for at this point.

CHANGES OBVIOUS FOUR WEEKS AFTER PACEMAKER

Four weeks into this new adventure in life I decided to take stock of the changes I have discovered since pacemaker surgery. Despite being confused this week with a sinus infection - at first, I thought the shortness of breath was the pacemaker going haywire- things have progressively improved.

I feel as if I am slowly coming back to life, although I

was nowhere near dead nor unhappy with life pre-pacer. On the contrary, I am blessed with wonderful people who make each day worthwhile and a God who is constantly with me. But my body feels remarkably better now, more energetic, and stable with a steady resting pulse.

In the last four weeks here are some of the things I have noticed or been able to do:

I am sleeping better.

I have walked up and down aisles at several small stores instead of going in and out as quickly as possible.

I went into two grocery stores for the first time in about two years and bought a few items.

I stood for 45 minutes during a workshop and had a blast (I am unsure how this happened, but I did have two bags of IV saline that day and held on to a wall, leaning occasionally).

I have been to Starbucks on several occasions, sat down and stayed for about an hour at a time, enjoying tea and the atmosphere. Three days after surgery I even made it to a Starbucks with a friend for about an hour.

I have begun to exercise again on a recumbent stationary bike. I began slowly; the longest I have gone is 35 minutes.

I went into a sporting goods store, stayed for about 20 minutes and proceeded to try on several coats before I found one to purchase.

I have had two sinus infections and while my blood pressure was labile, I was not as sick as in the past. My heart rate was much steadier, which felt good.

I walked my puppy a half mile.

I made it through daily Mass without having to leave.

I can stand longer before symptoms intrude.

These observations provide hope that the pacemaker is indeed a life-altering event and things will continue improving. When I go places, I feel like I have time to walk around, observe, and enjoy what I am doing rather than getting in and out before my body revolts. It is a liberating feeling.

I still crash, twice since surgery. The first time I pushed my body to the limit without resting and finally crashed hard, 17 days after surgery. I knew what I was doing but did not care. I wanted to see how far my body could go, without pacing. I stayed flat for two days and hopefully learned a lesson; despite the pacemaker I still have dysautonomia and need to pace energy. I believe I will probably need to repeat this lesson a few more times before it is imprinted on the brain.

I crashed a second time before the current sinus infection; likely due to illness. It is ok, I did not expect my nervous system to magically become repaired as a pacemaker cannot do this. But a new heartbeat rate feels good, and I am enjoying the freedom it is offering.

Hope is rising with each passing day.

PEOPLE DISAPPOINT REGARDLESS OF THE SITUATION

I had delusions that heart surgery would change behavior of others, but it was just that, delusions. People don't change unless they choose to change.

I have heard from three people directly, or indirectly,

about their anger towards me; anger since having pace-maker surgery.

Each is upset for the same reason; I chose to tell them of the pacemaker surgery hours after rather than before surgery. Most relatives and friends learned of the surgery after the fact. Perhaps others are angry, I don't know.

I have had amazing responses from many people in-cluding cards, compassion, dinners, phone calls and prayers. And then there are those who I thought would be supportive who have all but disappeared or expressed anger.

I defended myself to some, explaining part of the rea-soning behind my decision. I chose to keep surgery pri-vate for two reasons. The surgery scared me and the fewer people that knew the fewer that would make a big deal out of it, causing more anxiety for me, my husband and kids. And I wanted the kids to be protected from outside influences; they found out of the surgery just days before it occurred.

I realized something about those angry at this well-thought-out decision (which really was not a decision as I could not live forever with a heartbeat so low). This is not my problem, and some will never understand. It makes me extremely sad, but it is not about me, it is about them. None asked how it felt to get a pacemaker at the age of 49; how my husband or three children handled the situation or how difficult it was to make the choice to undergo sur-gery. None showed the tinniest bit of empathy towards the fact this was a game changer for us not them. For them it was simply why didn't you tell me about this?

I realized this is a selfish pattern. Most people don't change when others face life-altering circumstances. No matter how I had hoped (subconsciously) that this surgery would bridge the gap between us it will not.

What I can change is my expectations of people. I also need to continue to try to identify the amazing blessings in life: the people who love and care for me; my husband and children; an increased heartbeat aided by the pacemaker; God; our puppy Lucy; stars; good books; music; Starbucks iced tea; relationships; love and so much more. I have to remember that there is much to be thankful for in this world and not be brought down by those who cannot share in this joy.

Joy in essence is one of the great gifts in this world.

CARDIOLOGY APPOINTMENT REINFORCES DECISION

After a 300-mile drive and a three-hour wait I finally saw Dr. Blair Grubb for a follow up to pacemaker surgery.

Prior to seeing him, I had the pacemaker interrogated by Harry Hahn, R.N., cardiac EP Nurse, pacemaker clinic. I soon learned that an interrogation consists of placing an instrument over the heart to read the pacer. Adjustments are then made, which I felt. Harry explained he sped up the heart, which felt like flutters. He then turned down the voltage of the pacer; something common at the first post-operative visit.

I mentioned some pain and shortness of breath. I found out shortly thereafter these comments were passed on to Dr. Grubb, earning me an echocardiogram. Another hour wait ensued until I found out there was no fluid around the heart; all looked good. The pain was probably from the pacer settling under the skin.

I was finally put in a waiting room at 1 p.m. for the 11 a.m. appointment and at 2 p.m. saw the cardiologist. I discovered shortness of breath on stairs is a common complaint of pacemaker recipients. Dr. Grubb explained he could adjust the pacer to be more sensitive but we both agreed that would drive me crazy. As long as I knew why I was short of breath I could tolerate such.

The plan was to keep the pacemaker settings status quo as energy level and quality of life were improving. Blood pressure was a bit elevated, but the hope was that might settle down as I became accustomed to the higher heart rate. We agreed I would continue to exercise regularly and perhaps tweak the pacer settings after an upcoming Florida vacation. All-in-all it was a positive visit.

NEARLY FORGOT I HAVE A PACEMAKER IMPLANTED

Twenty-two weeks and a day. 145 days. Five months. I've had a pacemaker beating inside my chest long enough now to almost forget it is there. The scar is fading, the zapping pains minimal. The only reminders are when my son snuggles and puts his head on me the wrong way; I see the scar in the mirror; or feel the bump while applying cream.

I don't think about the pacer failing much anymore as it has worked steadily for five months. In fact, I'm sure it is doing its job as each time I take my pulse, which is rarely, it is usually in the low to mid 60's. Since the heartbeat cannot fall below 60 I surmise my pacer continues to work a large portion of the time. This is not a concern, just a fact, necessity and a confirmation that I made the correct decision to undergo the operation.

Quality of life has improved since the pacemaker. I still crash physically, as dysautonomia does not magically disappear. I think I have crashed about five-seven times since October. I find this minimal and amazing considering one of these events was the day after surgery and another was after traveling and vacationing in Florida for 10 days. I also lived through one of the coldest winters since being diagnosed, a time where I often saw my hands turning purple upon exiting the shower and having to hop quickly under an electric blanket; an occurrence that in the past would spiral into a crash.

Despite these difficulties, full-blown crashes- the kind that kept me flattened in bed with legs elevated, drinking Gatorade - were minimal.

The pacemaker has improved several other things in my life. These include I am able to sit at Starbucks for upwards of 45 minutes and visit or write. Prior to surgery, I was fortunate if I could last 20 minutes.

I can sit longer at church. Sometimes I can enjoy an entire mass, other times most of the service.

I continue to be able to exercise on an indoor bike 30-60 minutes every other day. My heart rate does not elevate too high but at least I can exercise.

I have been able to enjoy dinner out a few times; something I had not done in years.

I have driven upwards of 45 minutes, which is double the time prior to the pacer.

It is a fine line between knowing what I can do and pushing too far and suffering from the results of poor energy pacing. I continue to learn, live and enjoy the freedom that this life choice has afforded me. I am thankful that I have had this opportunity and will continue to enjoy wherever this journey goes.

SEARCHING FOR A NAME FOR PACEMAKER

I need a new name. It must be catchy but appropriate; fun but meaningful. I have been looking for the name for six months now, but it has not materialized. Others that travelled this road have created names but mine needs to be unique - to fit me perfectly. I know the name will come, but I am unsure when.

It is the six-month anniversary of having a pacemaker implanted below my collarbone. I had hoped to have a name by now but I don't. Regardless, the time has flown. I no longer think of my pacer daily. Occasionally, the scar itches or I will have to pull up my bra strap because it does not lie properly due to the bump of the pacemaker. Besides that I barely notice the pacemaker.

I am glad I decided to have the surgery, sooner, rather than later. Stamina for sitting, standing, walking and driving has improved considerably. People ask me if I am cured now, and I have to explain that no I still have dysautonomia which causes an array of physical problems. Having a heartbeat of at least 60 beats per minute, however, feels remarkable.

I have not been afraid to fall asleep because breathing

is shallow and heart rate too low since Oct. 9. That is a huge relief. That was a dreadful feeling that I became as accustomed to as possible; but at times was frightening. This feeling has been eliminated with the pacer.

I even tried out my pacemaker when the weather broke recently on a new 24-speed Trek bike. My heartbeat felt great - no skipped beats - and I pedaled five miles without symptoms. The second day I made four miles before the cold wind forced me to stop. The rides were great, but I failed to rest afterwards and both days crashed about three hours later. This produced the realization that I still must pace my energy. This is ok because life is better with a pacemaker - this much I am certain.

STABLE HEARTRATE FEELS COMFORTABLE

I have had a steady heartbeat for nine months. It hovers around 60-62 and feels strong and healthy. It is a beautiful thing; a reminder what modern science can do in today's world. I lived for about 25 years losing heart beats; first starting in the 60s as a norm and slowly becoming accustomed to operating at a typical 45-48 beats per minute.

I did not monitor my heartbeat on a regular basis but when a heart does not operate as well as it is supposed to one is intimately aware of such. I can still place two fingers on my neck and determine a heart rate within a couple of beats to near accuracy.

So on 10/9/13 I underwent a 90-minute operation to have a BIOTRONIK Evia pacemaker implanted under my collarbone with two leads attached to the heart. After an overnight stay at the University of Toledo Medical Center

- which extended into late afternoon the next day due to dysautonomia rearing its ugly head- I left the hospital. I headed 150 miles to a friend's house for four days of recovery before trekking home. Simple enough - well sort of except for all the emotional preparation before the surgery; physical and emotional healing afterwards.

I have a two-inch scar, a bump below my collar bone and the memories as a reminder.

Was it worth it? Definitely. It was a game changer.

Sure, I still have dysautonomia and all the annoying symptoms that go along with this disorder. But I am one of the "lucky" ones who has bradycardia instead of tachycardia. Bradycardia can be treated with a pacemaker designed specifically for dysautonomia patients thanks to my cardiologist Dr. Grubb and others. A pacemaker can't cure the disorder but can improve the quality of life.

This adventure has been a learning curve for the entire family. There have been emotions; fear, joy, apprehension, excitement, anger, happiness, defeat and victories. It has not been easy, and I still have dysautonomia—but I am thankful for the opportunity I was given.

Would I do it again—in a heartbeat? I am thankful to God first, and then Dr. Grubb.

INVENTORY TAKEN ELEVEN MONTHS POST-OPERATIVE

When I realized it was Sept. 9, I was surprised that 11 months had passed since a pacemaker was implanted.

I admit I don't think about the two-inch device daily, but I marvel at its benefits. Funny the 11-month anniversary was marred with two days of my body crashing; perhaps a not-so-subtle reminder that the pacemaker is not a cure all for a faulty autonomic nervous system.

I explained it recently that I am a "lucky one." Most with a form of dysautonomia called postural tachycardia orthostatic syndrome (POTS) have just that - tachycardia. Tachycardia is a higher than normal (60-100) heartbeat. My heart rate would not reach 100 even after an hour on an exercise bike or taking medicines to increase the rate. Rather it hovered in the 40s to 50s. As the POTS diagnosis suggests, when I stood, I would see a jump of 30 beats or more - which was unpleasant at best; causing a variety of symptoms.

Now the pacemaker works about 75-80 percent of the time to keep the heart rate at 62 beats or more per minute. We started at 60 beats and in July tried to increase to 65, but that produced a jumpy feeling. So after about five minutes Dr. Grubb decreased the rate to 62 and I have been at that rate since. To change the rate, a doctor or technician places an instrument over the pacemaker. The patient holds this while the medical person changes the settings through a computer-like instrument.

Sixty-two beats feel pretty good.

Dysautonomia lives, however. This includes nausea, pain, gastrointestinal problems, dizziness, headaches, blood pressure swings, the need for fluids, vitamins and medications and presyncope. I still can't stand upright long without symptoms, but there is added stamina.

I decided a year before my implant that I would live with dysautonomia the best I could. I would embrace life;

rejoice at the victories and do my best to overcome the defeats. Some days are not easy, but I persevere.

I am like the battery inside of me. It will eventually slow down and will need to be replaced. In the meantime, I will seek ways to recharge. And continue to live.

HEARTBEAT FEELS FABULOUS THANKS TO PACEMAKER

Heartbeat - one complete pulsation of the heart. The vital center of driving impulse. A brief space of time.

I added 20 extra heart beats a minute this year; 1,200 beats an hour; 28,800 beats a day; roughly 864,000 beats per month and 10,368,000 beats in the year since having a BIOTRONIK Evia pacemaker implanted on 10/9/13.

The pacemaker was a result of chronotropic incompetence - inability to sustain a steady heartbeat. In my case, despite the best efforts of medicine, my heart rate lingered in the low to mid 40s most of the time. The highest - after a hard bike ride immediately before surgery (as I was testing myself and my heart) - was about 98 beats per minute. This is very low for the exertion I put forth. I began losing beats slowly in my mid-20s (coincidentally after a bout of mononucleosis although I did not realize the connection for decades); had episodes in which it would slow, and I would feel badly; but at that time all tests were negative. In retrospect, I probably had mild signs of dysautonomia for decades. Eventually my heart rate became problematic enough for the pacemaker implant.

I love the extra beats. I don't physically feel the battery

inside me working, but I pace about 80 percent; meaning my natural heart rate cannot get to the lowest setting it is allowed on its own most of the time so the pacer kicks in. Structurally there is nothing wrong with my heart; rather the autonomic nervous system is faulty, causing the slowing heart rate.

What do I do with those extra beats? Live a fuller life.

The beats have allowed me more stamina - which is huge. The higher, steadier heart rate allows more energy and longer periods of being upright before rest is necessary.

In the year since my pacer, I feel like the shadow cast on my life has been replaced with brightness and color. I have been afforded more opportunities. Some experiences include:

- Traveled to Florida.
- Renewed wedding vows and celebrated with family and friends our 25th wedding anniversary.
- Went to my first 4th of July fireworks display in years.
- Returned to bike riding.
- Attended my nephew's wedding.
- Laughed, loved, lived, found joy.
- Celebrated my 50th birthday with a bike ride and a busy day with loved ones.
- Was spontaneous.
- Pushed the limits a little more.

- Saw the band the Goo Goo Dolls in concert twice.
- Attended more of our children's functions including doctor appointments and school events.

Sure, it has not all been easy; dysautonomia is a difficult condition to manage. And having a pacemaker took some adjustment. Most of the time, though, I don't even remember it is there.

There are occasions when I have a pain in my chest, or I am sick and worry that I might get an infection. And of course, there is that slight bump that sticks out below my collar bone.

I am thankful for the opportunity these extra heartbeats provide. I am doing the best to enjoy them, spend them wisely, happily and embrace life.

DOCTOR ASKS ADVICE ON HOW TO HELP OTHERS

My doctor asked me what factors helped me to improve my overall functioning. He wanted the information to utilize with another similar patient in his practice presenting with dysautonomia.

Medicines, God, doctors, writing, exercising, praying, running a HopeKeepers group and praying were the answers. And the pacemaker? he asked. Yes, and God I interjected.

Yes, I think I mentioned God or praying three or four times. And the best part was he didn't flinch as he understands the power of prayer. He then shared his frustration that he cannot reduce the amount of medications and vitamins I ingest daily, but we agreed they are necessary.

As I left his office and he wished me a good holiday season I walked with added confidence knowing he didn't want to see me again for four months - the longest time since chronic illness entered my life.

It has been a challenging journey filled with highs and lows. But the constant is faith. It has waned at times but continues to live within me despite obstacles.

I am fortunate to have a doctor who has been on this journey with me from the start. In fact I remember early on before we knew I had dysautonomia the doctor apologized for not yet diagnosing my autonomic dysfunction. With perseverance a diagnosis came; after much trial and error a treatment plan formed.

Recently, another primary care doctor in the practice encountered a patient with similar symptoms to me. Together with my doctor, she reviewed my records to decide on a treatment course. Perhaps the patient's journey to improved health will be shorter; it would be gratifying to know the knowledge learned through treating me will improve other's care. Regardless, ultimately God is in control.

PACEMAKER SETTINGS MAY BE INCORRECT

The pacemaker beating inside me for 17 months has provided a new outlook on life. I have more freedom and energy. It has allowed me a steady 62 bpm and recently my cardiologist and I agreed to bump it up to 64 bpm.

As part of the cardiology check-up, my doctor determines whether to change the pacers' settings. In addition to giving me two additional heartbeats, he increased the setting to be more sensitive to shifts in blood pressure. This will allow the heartbeat to rise more quickly when I stand as blood pressure drops (orthostatic hypotension). The hope is I will feel less symptomatic at the more sensitive setting.

I am not sure whether the setting is optimum. After three weeks, I am more fatigued and have felt some odd sensations. But I've been able to stand and walk slightly longer before becoming symptomatic. I wonder if I am not accustomed to the increased heart rate as bradycardia was a constant companion; and even with POTS I rarely went above 70 bpm. I have always been a bit stubborn and in this case I am grateful.

Stubborn - refusing to change your ideas

I will wait this out a bit longer and see what occurs. I will talk to my primary care doctor and seek his advice. I presume he will agree to wait and observe before making changes. The weather is finally warming, and the cold winter has been a huge challenge in dealing with dysautonomia. It is difficult to discern if this or something else is causing the added fatigue and other symptoms.

The beauty is I have this tiny piece of equipment that assists me in living a more fulfilled life; albeit different than when healthy. And now I will wait, embracing my stubbornness as I decide what is next.

I WOULD LIKE TO RIP PACEMAKER OUT OF BODY

I've had my pacemaker for 1.5 years. I recently wanted to rip it out of my chest.

Most of the time, however, I am happy to have this silver-dollar sized device.

It has performed well for me; pacing my heart nearly 80 percent of the time after autonomic dysfunction slowed the beat.

I didn't want to rip the pacemaker out of me because of malfunction. Rather I learned of the incompetence of some technicians who program the device. I also discovered that while someone may say they are trained to program a device, they actually may not have the proper expertise in dealing with dysautonomia. I must seek technicians or my cardiologist who are expertly trained; even if they are 300 miles from home. The technician I thought was knowledgeable was not; she programmed my pacemaker incorrectly resulting in me feeling very unwell. Once I discovered this, through conversations with Toledo, my husband drove 600-miles round trip in one day to get my pacemaker reprogrammed. I decided, after this, that I will only have my pacer settings changed by those who are truly knowledgeable. At this time I must travel to Toledo, Ohio.

In the last 18 months there have been ups and downs with my physical and emotional health. The day-to-day challenges of living with a chronic illness have been depressing at times. To think at 50 I have a device inside me that will need to be replaced every 10 years and could get infected, causing serious health problems, is daunting. The benefits outweigh the risks, however, and the added energy is priceless. I have been able to do things with my family that pre-pacer were impossible. And while it is nothing compared to the old life when I was healthy, at least there is improvement.

I can walk, bike, visit and even travel a bit now. Sure I have symptoms daily (actually hourly); but I make modifications and adjust. But I have more quality of life than I did 18 months ago. Everyone in my family is happier. My children have their mom back; maybe not fully but at least partly. And that is pretty good.

A LITTLE GRAVITY HUMOR

Finding humor despite the difficulties can be helpful. Here are two lists inspired by Sir Isaac Newton's theory of gravity.

TOP 10 WORST GRAVITY CHALLENGES

10. Movie theaters
9. Mountain driving
8. Human conveyor belts
7. Playground equipment
6. Aircraft ascent and descent
5. Flashing lights
4. Bumpy roads
3. Elevators
2. Amusement park rides
1. Tilt table tests

TOP 10 BEST SMALL BLESSINGS

10. Cool breeze of fresh air, after being in a hospital

9. Ice chips

8. Cold, wet cloth on face

7. Warm blanket

6. Steady arm to lean on

5. Called by name, good eye contact

4. "I believe you."

3. Popsicles

2. A hand to hold

1. Spoons.   SAR

TIPS FOR PREPARING FOR SURGERY

When faced with a medical procedure or surgery there are things you can do to help minimize complications and assert some control. These include:

- Talk to your doctor to have him/her explain the situation, risks and benefits. Have a list of questions written down so not to forget. Bring someone to the appointment, if possible, for a second set of ears.

- Have a plan for anesthesia. This may include meeting with that doctor ahead of time so he/she has an understanding of dysautonomia and how it affects you, and the complexities involved. Often the charge nurse is a helpful advocate.

- Have your primary care doctor's office request fluids before, during and after surgery, if agreed upon. Fluids are helpful for recovery.

- Discuss with your doctor plans for post-surgery recovery. Will you need home health services and if so have the doctor's office coordinate these services?
- Seek a second opinion.
- Remember to pace yourself after surgery. We often recover more slowly than healthier individuals.
- Give yourself permission to feel all the emotions that accompany surgery. These are normal and it is better to deal with the feelings than repress them. Seek support for varied feelings.
- When people offer help, take the assistance. Be specific on your needs which may include meals, transporting children, housekeeping, and other errands.
- Pack comfort items if staying in the hospital. These may include a favorite blanket, electronic devices and chargers, comfortable clothing and reading material.

DIARY QUESTIONS

Each person has a different treatment plan to treat dysautonomia or any other chronic illness. For Laura a pacemaker was necessary, although that is not the norm. What treatment plan has worked thus far for you?

If you have a medical device implanted, have you named it? And if so, what is the name and why?

What are five blessings you can note in your life?

What strategies have you found helpful in dealing with yet another medical test, diagnosis or procedure?

Chapter three: Having fun

"Hope anchors the soul."
—*Hebrews 6:19*

"Life is like a bicycle. To keep your balance you must keep on moving...."
—*Albert Einstein*

"Let them praise His name with dancing."
—*Psalm 149:3*

Sharon and I realized early on in our lives with chronic illness that we must still enjoy ourselves. There is no doubt this can be difficult; especially when dealing with medical crises or receiving one more diagnosis. We made conscious decisions to deal with the frustrations that come but also try to laugh at our situations. We have embraced humor. In fact, Sharon accompanied me to my autonomic testing at University Hospital Case Western in 2011. My husband dropped us at the entrance to make our way to neurology as he parked.

After insisting I could walk, despite being off medications, weak and wobbly, we stopped in the lobby for a rest. I decided to drink a protein shake - which Sharon discouraged- before going up on the elevator to the neurology floor.

Sharon also tried to convince me to go in a wheelchair, but I refused. So, she ran ahead to call the elevator, then waved me on. I stumbled to the elevator, and by the grace of God it was waiting for us. I would later discover Sharon pushed all the call buttons, yelled for me and hoped I did not drop while walking. We equate it, and us, to Lucy and Ethel in the television sitcom I Love Lucy.

Brain fog was heavy, and I could not think straight; Sharon helped me complete paperwork. We laughed as I continued to make little sense. About 20 minutes into the tilt table test, I burped immediately before passing out. I thought of Sharon when I regained consciousness and how she had warned me not to drink the shake. Thankfully I did not throw up.

Today if we mention the tilt table test, we both tell stories and laugh hard. My autonomic testing was a difficult day made better by friendship and humor. And that is the key; we still deal with our medical obstacles but find laughter and joy in our lives. I visit Sharon and her husband two to three times a year. We don't always get out of the house, but we sit, talk and laugh. Her friendship is truly a gift I cherish. Below are glimpses at enjoying life; despite dysautonomia.

A NEW BIKE TO EXPERIENCE PEDALING THROUGH LIFE

I purchased a 24-speed Trek hybrid bike. It is tidal green with a black seat. I pick it up soon and am excited. Temperatures are expected to reach 60; perfect weather to give the bike a spin.

Seven months ago, I never expected I would be in the

market for a new two-wheeler. I had nearly given up the idea of riding a road bike because dysautonomia robbed me of this pleasure. In fact, in the summer of 2010, it was bike riding that first gave me a clue that something was wrong. That summer, I could not ride more than five miles and twice I had to dive off the bike and get to the ground as I was dizzy, seeing spots and my heartbeat was crazy high. I was accustomed to riding 10-20 miles at a clip so I knew something was wrong. However, when I called my doctor's office the nurse chalked it up to dehydration. I knew something was not right.

I can still remember, years later, exactly where I was on the bike rides I aborted.

Never in my wildest dreams would I have known the medical journey that would follow. The days of long bike rides were over. In fact, the furthest I could go was five miles and eventually I stopped biking altogether. I switched to an exercise bike in which I worked up from five minutes daily to 45-60 minutes every other day.

Last September, I grabbed my old Specialized bike and gave it a spin a week before pacemaker surgery. I wanted to see what my heart would do and if my body could handle a ride. I pedaled five miles twice and learned two important facts:

1. I needed a pacemaker to sustain a heartbeat because my heart wasn't doing it on its own.

2. I was truly happy on a bike, even at five miles. I could stay upright for 30 minutes before becoming dizzy and nauseous, still sweat and feel my legs work. It felt fabulous.

At that moment I abandoned my plans for a recumbent trike bike and decided instead on a road bike. And I can't wait to try it out with a new, steady heartbeat. I don't know if I will be able to bike further, but I imagine it is a possibility. Regardless, I will bike; I will feel leg muscles burn; the wind on my face. I will smile, look around and enjoy the beauty that God has created. Since dysautonomia has entered my life I have said that I hope God has a bike for me in Heaven so I can go for a 20-mile ride at my leisure. I am getting a little piece of Heaven with this new bike. I can't wait to give it a spin.

EXCITED TO GO ON FAMILY BEACH VACATION

I will be on a Florida beach in less than two weeks. It will be our first family vacation in 4 1/2 years as dysautonomia stole vacations from us. We are taking a huge leap of faith and hoping I tolerate traveling.

We head to Florida for a 10-day vacation. It is an early 25th wedding anniversary celebration for my husband and I and we decided to take the kids along. Our family needs a vacation; a time to regroup, breathe, smell the sea air and relish the ocean calm after a crazy 2013.

We faced five surgeries in 2013 - three for my mother-in-law, one for my daughter and one for me.

After surviving back surgery, we almost lost my husband's mother to a bowel obstruction which poisoned her systems. Months of rehabilitation and an additional surgery finally brought her back. Then we watched our daughter tear her second ACL while playing softball. To hear her cry in anguish and frustration as she was carried off the softball field was heartbreaking but what was more distressing was knowing immediately she had just done to her right knee what she had done to her left one 12 months earlier. She knew too and was crying both in pain and from the realization she would face surgery; eight months of rehabilitation and no sports again for the better part of a year.

In August I was told it was time for a pacemaker. Sure, I could wait but bradycardia was not improving through medications and my surgeon was offering hope that quality of life could improve with surgery. We both believed a pacemaker might even make the vacation more enjoyable. On October 9 I had a pacemaker implanted.

Five weeks later we prepare for vacation. First, I head to Toledo to get the pacemaker checked. Nine days later we hop on a plane. Sounds simple enough but not really. There is planning, packing, pacing and praying. There is a loose plan in place in case I need fluids while away; hopefully if that is the case the emergency room will understand dysautonomia.

I plan to board the plane first to secure a front seat with additional leg room. That way I can put my feet up as necessary; otherwise, I am sure to become symptomatic more quickly.

Once in Florida I will rest for at least 24 hours while the remainder of the family explores. By day two I hope to be ready for some fun. I admit that all the planning and pacing is frustrating. Sometimes it is lonely; I feel left out of things. If I don't plan, however, life can quickly deteriorate. And if I crash on vacation, I could miss upwards of three days.

I can't push my body on this trip. I need to listen carefully to signs of dehydration and fatigue. I must rely on my husband and the kids to be ok without me at times and I have to realize I can't do everything. I will try to relish what I can experience, rather than become saddened with what I can't perform.

After all, I am going to Florida, to the ocean. I may see dolphins, put my toes in the sand, find sand dollars and breathe the amazing sea air. The ocean is peaceful and calming and makes my soul come alive.

December 2, 2010, I woke up with a flu. It was a flu that I later found out most likely caused permanent damage to my autonomic nervous system kicking dysautonomia into high gear within the next few months. That flu changed my life.

Three years later I am going to embrace the anniversary by savoring our last day on the Gulf of Mexico; as close to paradise as possible with people I love.

FLORIDA SUN IS GREAT PRESCRIPTION FOR RELAXATION

I am basking in the Florida sun - day five of a 10- day vacation 4.5 years in the making.

I never anticipated it would take so long to go on vacation after our April 2009 Outer Banks, NC trip when I was healthy; but dysautonomia got in the way of life and postponed a bit of fun for a stretch. My husband and I realized we were coming up on our 25th-wedding anniversary in December and decided nothing was going to stop us from celebrating, not even a chronic condition. So in June, plans were set for a Thanksgiving beach vacation. We decided to skip our actual December 30 anniversary because the winter cold leaving Buffalo, NY would likely have adverse effects on my health. I cannot tolerate extreme temperatures; too hot or cold.

In August, when my cardiologist threw in the mix that I should get a pacemaker sooner rather than later, the decision was made to have it implanted prior to the vacation in hopes the trip would be more enjoyable. And it has. I am walking daily at the ocean's edge while looking for seashells. I have not walked this far since pre-dysautonomia.

I still need to rest daily as my body is achy; there are headaches and nausea, but functioning is remarkably better. I have even been out shopping and to dinner.

It is so peaceful at the ocean, actually paradise. We are happy, calm and filled with joy. There is no schedule and the view from the room as we awake or fall asleep is the ocean. It is easy to become accustomed to this life. I am thankful we took this leap of faith and gave traveling another chance.

BIKING EXPERIENCE BEST PART OF DAY

I road eight glorious miles on my 24-speed Trek today. It was humid and sweat dripped down my face and back. It was an amazing feeling as I typically don't sweat much due to autonomic dysfunction.

I didn't think I would ever feel my leg muscles work hard or heart pound quickly again; but God has restored this gift and I choose to savor it. Biking outdoors is remarkably better than using a stationary bike. My legs are the pilot; they direct the bike and me, taking us our distance. They determine speed, miles and terrain; allowing me to see the beautiful land, sky, people, buildings and nature.

Today's goal was five miles, but stubbornness stretched it to eight. The ride included a nine-minute rest at five miles after I began feeling foggy, numb in the hands with shoulder/neck pain - all symptoms that blood is pooling in the legs, depriving my brain of oxygen, and I need to get off my bike. Thankfully putting feet up and drinking Gatorade allowed me to continue on the ride.

It has been eight months since pacemaker surgery, and I never imagined I would be able to ride this far again. I am so thankful for this gift, which I don't take for granted. Each time I strap on a helmet, put on biking gloves, set the odometer and climb on the bike I marvel at the fact I am going out for a ride. I thank God for these opportunities. I smile while biking until my breath gets labored and I grimace, but the spirit smiles nonstop.

My challenge is to continue to enjoy the rides and try to recover. Today's ride, despite drinking fluids during and after, resulted in almost immediate diarrhea. Fluid loss is an enemy to someone with dysautonomia as dehydration is a constant threat. Added salt and fluids are necessary after biking. The challenge is whether I recover from this ride more quickly than the last "long" ride. I am pushing more fluids this time in hopes of a better outcome.

Regardless, I made a choice. I will enjoy the rides; try not to fear the crashes; embrace the present; and thank God for this amazing gift - the gift of biking once again.

HAVING FUN WORTH EXHAUSTION AFTERWARDS

I spent the last two days at home, often flat, with feet up. I reclined, slept, read, watched Netflix, listened to music, and got up occasionally. I drank a lot of fluids and took extra salt tablets. Nausea, headaches and light headedness were near constant companions and driving was out of the question. But I was happy, joy filled. I did question myself for a moment but knew if I stayed the course of fluids and rest I would eventually recover. And I knew the reason I felt so badly, and it was well worth it.

I completed a 10-mile charity bike ride, the Ride for Roswell 2014, in 80-degree weather. It took a little more than an hour, due to the incredibly jam-packed start until my husband and I found our groove. We also needed to stop at five miles to rest. I knew resting was part of the plan as after about five miles symptoms arise. If I don't stop I would be unsafe on a bike. After about 10 minutes of resting and fluids I was ready to continue the route.

I wore colorful compression stockings that looked like peace signs painted all over the legs. They garnered several comments from supporters. Some riders thought my legs were tattooed until they were close enough to realize I was wearing socks.

The ride was glorious. After a four-year hiatus from this event due to dysautonomia I finally knew this was the year to give the ride a chance. Two months ago, I came up with a plan. And after my doctor initially expressed his concern and shock, he gave me his blessing. He joked that he would be away for that weekend if anything were to occur.

I practiced biking outside slowly building up the miles until I was ready for the ride. I knew I could cover the 10 miles if my body cooperated, and with dysautonomia that is a big unknown. I had my husband with me for safety, along with a helmet, fluids and an eight-month-old pacemaker beating inside me. The joy of beginning the ride, knowing I had raised a large sum of money for cancer research, and then completing the course is indescribable. It was a huge personal victory and worth the physical crash that ensued.

I don't know how long I will be able to bike outside, but each day I strap on my bike helmet I thank God for the second chance I have been granted.

EMERGENCY ROOM VISIT DOESN'T HALT CHARITY RIDE

Two days after my first Emergency Department (ED) visit since dysautonomia joined my life, I road 10 miles in a charity bike ride for the second consecutive year; the Ride for Roswell 2015. The hope of riding was first dashed when I spent six hours in the ED receiving three bags of fluids. Blood tests showed low iron but thankfully a transfusion was not necessary. Instead, my primary doctor prescribed large doses of oral iron.

I rested the next day, increased fluid intake and tried to admit the ride was in jeopardy. By nightfall I had not given up and packed my belongings in preparation for a rainy event.

Of course, my brain had other ideas. Two hours before the venture, I awoke with an ocular migraine. I tried to pretend my vision was not deteriorating but within 10 minutes I had a full-blown light show in my eyes. I knew if I took migraine medication my body would turn heavy, and chances of riding would evaporate. Instead, I took over-the-counter medicine; showered with crazy lights flashing in my eyes; dressed and rested. Thirty minutes later, I was left with a slight headache, tiredness and nausea. But I was not giving in to these symptoms; I could see, stand and was going to head to the ride with my husband in the driver's seat.

We drove in silence as I drank fluids, elevated feet, rested and prayed. Upon arrival I was determined to continue. While waiting for the event to begin, I sat on a bench first, then the ground as standing for those 10 minutes would cause symptoms.

It was 60 degrees outside and as the ride began so did light rain. The rain turned heavy as my husband and I joined thousands in pedaling for cancer research. Finally, we were off, passing spectators including cancer survivors and others cheering us on. The ride went smoothly, despite downpours. We checked our brakes often, pedaled a bit slower (one hour for 10 miles) and talked as we enjoyed each other's company. Afterwards we benefited from perks of raising more than $2,000 including lemon chicken, fruit and a variety of sports drinks.

Typically, I get lightheaded, nauseous and experience a headache on rides and need to stretch and hydrate. Despite the unpredictable, summer weather, I road straight through on this day, with perhaps a 120-second stop to secure another Gatorade.

Crossing the finish line was euphoric. I told my husband that I wish he could taste the sweetness of this ride as we pedaled the last half mile. When we crossed the finish, I grabbed his hand and we pedaled triumphantly together.

About 45 minutes later, I knew we better head out; once to the car I stripped the wet clothes off and changed. I was cold and a bit foggy.

My stomach was kind enough to wait until I returned home to explode. I took a quick, hot shower and dressed in warm clothes. Four hours later I awoke feeling slightly better. My limbs were a bit heavy and heart rate elevated but I knew I accomplished a goal.

The aftereffects were well worth the joy.

ROLLER COASTER METAPHOR IS FITTING

I hate roller coasters.

That was my 2011 Facebook status after a dismal cardiology appointment when I had hoped to receive effective treatment for dysautonomia but rather was told I was not "sick enough" for the arrogant doctor to assist. Granted, he did me one favor and referred me to Dr. Blair Grubb who eventually would help turn the medical situation more hopeful.

This roller coaster analogy continues to fit my medical and emotional state of chronic illness and I have always, always hated roller coasters.

Today, I am faced with apprehension, excitement and frustration; a norm lately when big events occur. There is a huge family gathering - the 25th anniversary mass and reception for my brother as a Roman Catholic priest. The church will be packed; I will see cousins who traveled from as far away as Arizona and Massachusetts and other family and friends I love. I am sure it will be a beautiful mass.

I think of my parents; my mom so proud of her son 25 years ago on his ordination day. And my dad I am sure watching from Heaven then and now; his own brother studying to become a priest until World War II cut his life and dreams short.

Twenty-five years ago, I was young, full of hope and healthy. I was newly married just three weeks in and awed at the site of my brother lying prostrate on the alter in front of the bishop, family, friends and God, proclaiming his life to service. Back then I did not have to worry if I slept poorly, had a migraine headache and a horrible week both emotionally and physically. All these factors challenge me today as I pray for a body that cooperates enough to enjoy this celebration. In 1989 I wouldn't have thought twice about any of this.

Roller coasters go up and down, oftentimes rather quickly with little warning. Sort of like life. Sure, there are plateaus, and yes some excitement is necessary. But today I wish I could hop in the shower without worrying whether simple changes in temperature will cause head pressure or presyncope feelings. I wish I could sit in the church and afterwards visit, walk around at the reception and stand as long as necessary. I would like to be normal today. Like I was 25 years ago. Just for today.

CLASSMATE ASKS "WHAT'S YOUR STORY?"

I sat down at my 30-year high school reunion determined to have fun. It was 80-degrees that summer night and heat was an enemy. I knew I'd need to drink a lot of Gatorade and water, elevate feet and hope. I rested most of the day, drank extra fluids, prayed and was ready to enjoy myself.

I looked more relaxed than most as dysautonomia makes it impossible for me to sit normally. Instead, I elevate my legs to keep blood pressure more stable. Sometimes I use two chairs, other times I just wrangle my legs on one. Early on that evening, two people approached, a husband and wife. I remember the young man as a skinny, kind kid in high school. He had grown into a hulking, handsome man. The first thing out of his mouth was "so what is your story?"

"What do you mean?" I asked.

He had read a little of my restministries.com writings on the internet and wanted to know more. Restministries is a Christian ministry devoted to supporting those with chronic conditions. I told him and his lovely wife about dysautonomia and my faith in God. He interjected that he was a two-time cancer survivor and would never have persevered without God. He was blessed every day and the hardest part of his struggles was seeing what it had done to his family.

It was as if nothing else mattered in the huge tent full of classmates, some I had not seen since attending the previous reunion 10 years earlier, others since graduation. We were in our own little world then, talking about God, illness, and the blessings during our struggles. This was about 20 minutes into the night and I could have left then and been happy. Without my illness I would never have had the opportunity to encounter this generous couple; hear their story; and share experiences. I am convinced God brought us together.

The night progressed and I had the pure pleasure of seeing old friends I had not seen in so long. I reconnected with one of my dearest friends who I lost touch with after my wedding. We vowed to stay in touch this time.

Late in the evening someone came up and saw me stretched out on two chairs. She asked if I had an ankle injury. I explained why I sit oddly, and she said her husband had a brain tumor. What, I thought? We talked about his struggles; how it changed the family system; his treatment; how God has blessed their lives and how they rely on faith to survive. Wow, what an amazing conversation, all because I had my legs elevated.

I left the reunion happy for several reasons. What was most profound was my experience would have been much different if I did not have a chronic illness. Strange how life works that way at times.

OBSTACLES ASIDE, SOUTH CAROLINA TRIP A SUCCESS

I recently completed a trip in which I flew with my daughter to South Carolina to visit friends I had not seen in several years. Health problems of the friend and I prevented us from getting together sooner, like we had done in the past.

Traveling can be difficult for anyone but having a chronic condition makes it even more difficult. In my case the illness is invisible - except when I turn ghost white when I come close to passing out and need to dive to the floor. Invisible illnesses, I have learned, can cause extra challenges while traveling.

On our way down to S.C. I pre-boarded with a medical pass. While I did not hear the women behind me in the wheelchair, my daughter reported to me that she audibly complained that this line was for handicapped people only. I considered saying something to her but decided God would prefer I stay quiet. However, when the flight attendant encouraged me to sit in the third row instead of first for more leg room, I explained I needed the first row so I could elevate my feet; so not to pass out. The woman gawked at me; perhaps understanding that I indeed have physical limitations. It turned out the employee and I both had pacemakers, so we compared brands.

On the way home I was ready to pre-board but was left standing as the attendant passed me up for eight people in wheelchairs: despite an explanation of my needs. By the time I entered the plane symptoms were roaring, as standing makes me ill. But I should have trusted God, and did thank Him, as a front-row seat was still available. On the next flight I explained my neurological condition ahead of time and the kind employee let me board first. I sent a letter of complaint to the airline, explaining how ignoring my need to pre-board regardless of whether I was in a wheelchair or not was discriminatory. I asked them to review their policies with their employees. I also praised the gentleman attendant who helped me on the connecting flight.

I don't respond well to flying; my body feels like it is on a roller coaster the entire flight. Anything I can do to alleviate more problems is helpful. But I realized people with invisible illnesses can be discriminated against. Thankfully God was with me while I traveled.

SABRES' HOCKEY HOME OPENER A THRILL

I walked into the Buffalo Sabres' National Hockey League arena on 10/9/14 and breathed deeply. I glanced around and saw blue and yellow balloons and smiling people wearing hockey jerseys. I heard the noise of happy crowds. I was there again, finally, after a long absence. I could not have been happier; thrilled actually.

It was my first Buffalo Sabres' game in four years, on the one-year anniversary of pacemaker surgery. It was the season and home opener for the Sabres and two of my kids, my husband and I had 200-level table seats, with waitress service, compliments of the Sabres. The seats allowed me to stretch and alleviate the symptoms of dysautonomia that come from my legs being down and immobile.

Perhaps everything was just a little bit sweeter; from the beautiful family singing the National Anthem in harmony; to the turkey club sandwich; to the vice-president of ticketing stopping by to see how we were enjoying ourselves; because I hadn't been able to attend a game for so long. And it was glorious, despite the 3-1 loss.

To head up on the elevator; step off and only have to walk a short distance to our seats was a treat in itself. No escalators or stairs to deal with; and only a short elevator ride prevented me from dealing with nausea and dizziness.

The seats were perfect. They were moveable which allowed me to stretch and elevate my legs consistently; helping to keep symptoms at bay. Fatigue set in but by that time the game was nearly complete and my family tired. They needed to get up early for school the next day. I did not disappoint anyone; in fact, I didn't even suggest leaving slightly early, one of the kids did. I am glad we left as energy had evaporated.

Even exiting the arena, I was enamored by the sights and sounds I observed. From the bronze statue of Sabres' French Connection line lit up in the dark to the pictures of current Sabres on the wall outside the arena, the place screamed of hockey.

While the game's outcome was disappointing, there was a feeling of festivity in the air from the moment we stepped into the building until we entered our car. We all knew this was a victory for me and our family, to again be able to attend a game. I have been a fan for about 40 years; have attended games since the late 1970s. We have had season tickets for about nine years. To give up going to live games was difficult; to get back for the home opener wonderful.

Now we have to devise a plan in which I can sit in our season ticket seats and find a location to stretch my legs as needed. That is next on my to-do list. Thankfully the vice-president of ticketing is willing to accommodate this goal by walking around the arena some quiet day to locate just the spot.

For now I am going to revel in the memory of that October 9th night; and be thankful for the gift of attending the game.

DRIVING PERMIT FOR DAUGHTER MUST WAIT A DAY

Our 16-year-old daughter wanted to get her driver's permit. Simple enough; hop in the car and go. Not so easy for someone with a chronic illness, as preplanning and communication are vital.

She asked at 1 p.m., three hours before the New York State Department of Motor Vehicles (DMV) closed for the day and one hour after I had used up an exorbitant amount of energy on errands. These errands were for a family birthday party that night for her and included stopping at three stores. Between recovering from a sinus infection, being in a car for an hour and shopping, I was tired; so much so that I had no idea how to get my daughter to the DMV. I said no, became disappointed, sad and frustrated, and cried.

I cried because I was angry my body was not like most

other moms who did not have to weigh everything they did to decide whether they could make it through to completion without dropping. I cried because I am sick of chronic illness and want the old me back; the one that went nonstop for hours on end without thinking of energy or stamina.

I cried because I worry what this does to my kids; not having a mom who can just do normal things like go with her daughter for a driving permit.

Getting a permit is a rite of passage. Not the first one I missed and not the last, I am sure, because of this dreadful diagnosis.

But something remarkable happened. My daughter saw me upset and said "mom, it is ok, this is not your fault."

After thanking her for this kindness I had to marvel at her empathy. She really did understand this had nothing to do with my want, because every ounce of me wanted to take her to the DMV. Rather it was a pure need, I needed to stay home, and she understood.

Our daughter earned her permit the following morning and I had the pleasure of driving with her. She drove pretty well.

NEW JOB MAY BE CHAUFFEUR TO THREE KIDS

I have done a lot of driving recently. Raising two teenagers and a 10-year-old often requires carting them to sporting events, school functions and appointments. Add to the list the appointments I have with my primary care doctor and specialists and sometimes the monthly planner can look as busy and filled as someone who works.

I am amazed at the fact I can now drive 30-45 minutes instead of the 10 minutes during the early stages of illness. I give credit first to God for this advancement - as without His intervention I could never have found a medical team which offered a pacemaker and medications to improve quality of life.

I must admit, however, driving to appointments is exhausting. I have found a few things have made life a little easier while managing this schedule.

I bring my iPad with me for the times I must wait. This way I can read and if there is free internet service can utilize different sites.

I always have fluids and a small snack on hand as these are necessary.

I bring daily medications in a pill container everywhere.

A good book is helpful (also available on iPad).

I wear a medic-alert bracelet in case of emergency and have a cell phone and identification with me.

I bring or wear a sweater, regardless of the weather as waiting rooms have varying temperatures. Gloves are also a constant as my hands are often the first body part to become cold.

I have to put my feet up. I have learned not to allow pride to get in the way and instead find a place in the room to recline; otherwise, symptoms will quickly occur making the visit unmanageable.

With some preparation, outings while dealing with chronic illness are more successful.

MOVING TO NEW HOME IMPOSSIBLE WITHOUT HELP

Packing, moving, unpacking, settling, adjusting - all part of moving to a new home. This is the third home we have purchased in our marriage; our fifth residence. For two of the kids, it is their third home, for our youngest his second.

We chose this house for several reasons; the layout is good for all of us. With two bedrooms and a bathroom on both the first and second floors we are spread out enough for privacy. In addition, with my physical needs the first-floor bedroom is easier for preserving energy as I don't need to climb stairs daily.

We also like the location in the village. There are sidewalks for walking and riding bikes and stores and restaurants are a short walk or drive. The kids' schools are also less than a mile from home.

Driving back and forth, even when it was only six miles roundtrip, became tiresome for me. This move should really help with conserving energy, a premium I often cannot control.

There have been some bumps in the move. Added stress has increased anxiety. Tensions have risen. A cold virus seems to have hit most of the family.

But all in all we are adjusting to our life change and the added work was well worth the effort.

TIPS FOR MOVING

Moving can challenge your body. The stress of packing, moving and unpacking can be huge. And if the move is geographically far, it can be more challenging. Here are suggestions to help with the process.

- Throw out items and donate what you can.
- Get help moving. If someone offers help take it. Ask for help. We often have a difficult time asking, but help is necessary.
- Hire teens or movers to assist
- Pack over months not days or weeks.
- Do not move furniture or boxes, leave that to the healthier people.
- Stay hydrated.
- Eat snacks.
- Sign legal papers ahead of time if possible.
- If money/figures are involved, make sure someone you trust can review.
- Find a set place in house for all keys to stay organized.
- Take your time unpacking. The job does not need to be finished immediately. Have someone set up and make your bed the first night; put soap and towels in bathroom and order take-out for dinner.

HOLIDAY TIPS

Holidays can stress a healthy body. Having a chronic condition can throw a curve into holiday plans. Here are some suggestions for dealing with and enjoying the holidays.

- Streamline. Pick three favorite cookies, not 10 varieties, to bake. Or order cookies from the local bakery.

- Accept whatever help is offered.
- Do not fuss about the exact date/day of the holiday. We use 'the octave' approach. We celebrate anywhere near the eight days before or after the actual date.
- Make a to-do master list. Subdivide it into clean, do-ahead. For example: set table, address labels, gifts and mailing. Food preparation: plan menu, make list, order specialty items, shop. Some items can be purchased on-line.
- Order to-go food at the local supermarket or restaurant if cooking is too challenging and ask guests to bring a certain item.
- Your home does not need to look immaculate.
- Pick your favorite display.
- Nap.
- Gifts: give gift cards. Hire a teen to wrap or use gift bags. Shop online.
- Find one present that you can give to several people.
- Ask friends that you typically buy for if they would like to spend time together instead, and only exchange gifts at birthdays.
- Keep a holiday journal. Jot down menus, repeats, or never repeat.
- Put your feet up. It is ok to have your blanket on the couch. If necessary, sneak away for a few minutes to lie flat in a quiet room.
- Use a smaller plate. Gastric problems make a big meal difficult to digest.

- Drink plenty of fluids and don't forget medications.
- Stay away from alcohol as it is a vasodilator and can lower blood pressure.
- Nap beforehand. It is acceptable to excuse yourself early or tell hostess that your time will be limited to just desserts.
- Steer conversations away from medical issue. Instead ask for a recommendation for a favorite television show, movie, author or book series.
- If you typically attend a church service, consider watching online.
- Pray. Keep mindful of the sick and those who have to work the holidays.
- Get leftover containers; make meals to go. This way you only have enough food you know will be eaten, not wasted.
- Put someone in charge of music, filling drink orders, taking coats, setting food out, and clearing dishes.

TRAVELING TIPS

Traveling can be fun but taxing on our bodies. Here are some suggestions for successful vacationing.

- Stay within one color palette of clothing, this allows pieces to be interchangeable.
- Be ready for rain or cold, both of which throw off temperature stability. Have a sweater/jacket for the cool air conditioning in some buildings. Dress in layers.

- Roll into one parcel all the clothes to be worn for one day.
- Put aside items for bathing including flip flops, towels and toiletries.
- Wear sunscreen. Bring hand sanitizer.
- Fill pill sorter for entire week; take cell phone photos of labels. This never leaves your reach. Ditto for your cell phone charger.
- Bring flannel blanket rolled with pajamas and slippers.
- Bring powdered salty drinks to always have some on hand.
- Keep mints, small snacks and medications in your bag with you.
- Always book one to two days prior to special events so you have time to rest up for the big occasion. I learned the hard way, and missed seeing Mama Mia on Broadway, New York City.
- Sleep, sip fluids and keep salty snacks and protein bars on hand.
- Always tell someone where you are going. If driving, review the route ahead of time and give yourself extra time for stops to elevate legs and rest.
- Have cash in small denominations.
- Update your Medic Alert bracelet information prior to departure.
- When choosing a plane seat, get an aisle seat so you can stretch legs better. Get to your seat when they announce: "If traveling with small children, or

if you need extra time." You can also ask to pre-board. Do not select an exit row, because they will move you if you are physically unable to open emergency door and assist with evacuation.

- To lessen nausea in a cab, look at a fixed point. Stay buckled. On a train hold on to a pole and take a seat as soon as someone gets up; some coaches have handicapped assessable seating.
- If in a car, stop every hour or so to stretch.
- Bring your handicapped car tag with you.
- Above all, stay hydrated and warm. Carry gloves in your bag to keep hands warm. Try not to touch your face because you may have touched a public surface which may spread germs.

TIPS FOR HANDLING EXTREME TEMPERATURES

Living in northeast Ohio, I am exposed to seasonal temperature variations: from summer's high 90's to winter's -10 degrees, not considering wind chills. I am unable to tolerate these extremes, nor any day in which there is a 30-degree temperature shift, or impending storm. The drop in barometric pressure makes my head feel like a dancehall, sparkly, ceiling ball.

The following adaptations have been successful:
- Stock-up. I plan as much stocking up during the spring and fall as possible. This includes all food staples, freezer food, and non-perishables. This helps reduce the times I am venturing outside

when I cannot tolerate temperature extremes. When I shop, I only bring in the perishables, my husband retrieves the rest of the bags.

- Limit stops to two stores. Temperature extremes really zap stamina. Or order food delivery service or drive-up service so you do not need to enter store.

- Plan. I have developed the skill of shopping online for gifts ahead of birthdays and try to have all preparations ready for send-out gifts a month ahead of time.

- In winter, warm car ahead of time. In summer, cool down car before driving.

- Clothes: I wear linen, silk and cotton, and layer clothing. These materials breathe and do not make me itch. I always have gloves and scarf in the car as needed.

- Fleece blanket, warmed in dryer if needed, folded with short sides together is helpful.

- Add additional blanket, so that when you crawl inside there is one beneath you and two on top.

- Calendar: I plan as many appointments with doctors, dentist, hairdresser etc. as I can in the milder seasons of spring and fall. When invitations arrive during summer or winter, it makes it less likely that I will be able to attend, and I try to make the hostess aware of my restrictions.

- When in this hibernation mode, I try to view it as an opportunity. I plan to learn one new skill, such as knitting, reading books, assembling scrapbooks that have been aching for completion and taking on-line course. I also try to stay in touch with friends.

DIARY QUESTIONS

What activities do you still perform that bring you joy?

What new activities have you discovered?

Exercise is often suggested despite the difficulty it presents. What is your exercise plan? And if you don't have one, what is one activity you could try to strengthen your body?

What tips can you provide for traveling and celebrating holidays when energy is at a premium?

Chapter four: Life and death

"All that live must die, passing through nature to eternity."
—William Shakespeare

"The life of the dead is placed in the memory of the living,"
—Marcus Tulius Cicero

"You can't do anything about the length of your life, but you can do something about its width and depth."
—Evan Esar

"In the end, it's not the years in your life that count. It's the life in your years."
—Abraham Lincoln

It is natural to experience fear when dealing with chronic conditions. We take several medications; our hearts beat erratically and have blood pressure readings that may jump up or down just from movement. No wonder we sometimes think about death. As we know, everyone dies. Preparation is not a bad idea. Make your plans, discuss them, then stop. No need to perseverate on death.

WILL DYSAUTONOMIA CAUSE AN EARLY DEATH?

None of us knows our life expectancy. No one knows their fate; how we will die, when, where. What we do know is that we all die, and life involves struggles, some visible, other's invisible.

While living with chronic illness, I have pondered if life will be shortened. I imagine an earlier death will be an indirect side effect of ingesting 28 pills (six prescriptions and a multitude of vitamins) daily or the added salt consumed to help keep upright. Without salt and Adderall, blood pressure dives and I experience presyncope. Presyncope is that dreadful feeling that I will pass out at any instance. Proper balance of fluids and medications helps keep presyncope somewhat at bay. Yet I wonder what ingesting all these things does to a body.

What I have learned thus far is worrying is futile. Fear is worthless. Thinking too much about death does not help one celebrate life. Each day is a gift with challenges. When dealing with dysautonomia, changing positions can become tricky. Standing or sitting may change blood pressure and heart rate and make it feel as if I am riding a roller coaster at times.

But there are ups and downs in everyone's journey, even if a body is not revolting. Life is both a challenge and a gift.

I find it more helpful to try to live day to day than fret about living with this disorder for decades. Thinking I could have symptoms for 30-plus years is daunting at best. Taking one day at a time is viable. I can awake each morning and thank God for another day. I hope for the best and when my body revolts I will adjust to what is occurring. Perhaps this includes increasing fluids, resting or elevating feet. And when I become discouraged because my body revolted, I need to change thoughts and get back on track. It is not always an easy or quick fix.

But my body is the way it is. The autonomic nervous system will heal only if a miracle occurs. And none of us are guaranteed anything. So living the best life is the only choice.

IS PRE-PLANNING FOR DEATH NECESSARY OR MORBID?

After spending 30 minutes scrubbing the grime off my parents' headstone, dirt that had most likely deposited since my mother's name was added to the stone years ago, I sat in the stillness of the surroundings.

I have often found this cemetery peaceful. Perhaps it is because as a youngster my dad would take me to Holy Cross Cemetery in Lackawanna, NY to plant flowers at relative's graves. I don't remember getting my hands dirty, rather I recall dad buying me a Henry's hamburger and fries. I'd have lunch, talk and play while he did the manual labor. It is a fond memory of time spent with dad.

It is natural, I believe, that I enjoy bringing a potted plant to St. Peter and Paul Cemetery in Hamburg, NY each year and placing it at my parents' grave. Sometimes the kids tag along, oftentimes I play music and pray.

I have found comfort here for years. Dad's been buried since late 1976; mom June 2000. I remember the day she died. I stopped by the cemetery before heading up to

Roswell Park Cancer Institute, Buffalo, NY, to be with her when life support ended. We knew it was probably her last day and I went for a long bike ride before driving in a huge thunderstorm to get to her. It was as if the universe knew how sad we were that day.

A pink geranium planted the week prior to mom's death had bloomed beautifully that June day at the cemetery. Funny, a few days after my day died in December 1976, my brother found blooming geraniums in our laundry room. Since then, I have chosen this flower to plant in honor of Dad; and they often stay hearty far beyond their season.

The day before mom's burial, I dug up that pink geranium so we could replant it once she was in her final resting spot. The morning of her funeral, I again biked to the cemetery to check out the surroundings. Biking was the only thing that gave me some solace during this time of great loss.

Years have passed and at times there is grief, but mostly there are memories and the knowledge of the love my parents had for one another and us.

And the thought entered my mind - will I be buried in this cemetery? If so, do we need to find a spot soon or can we wait? When I asked my husband, he could not fathom the idea of looking for a plot. And since one of us wants cremation and the other burial that makes for some interesting negotiations.

As I walked through sections of the cemetery, I envisioned a final resting place and wondered where I would choose. There are many spots left but surely that won't last. Then I wondered am I thinking this way because of my age; I will turn 50 soon. Or is it more likely the fact I have a chronic illness? While chronic illness does not mean terminal, I have wondered whether dysautonomia will hasten death.

No doctor has told me life expectancy is shorter now, but I have to wonder with all the changes I go through daily. Thankfully I had life insurance prior to diagnosis so that is not a concern for my family.

I guess for now the best I can do is embrace this life; trust God and enjoy what adventures I encounter.

ATTEMPTING TO STAY AS HEALTHY AS POSSIBLE

I am biking for life, my life.

After the cardiologist said my diagnosis is probably Pure Autonomic Failure (PAF) I realized a few things.

There are some parallels between that diagnosis and the fatal form of dysautonomia, Multiple Systems Atrophy (MSA). I can't worry whether I am heading down that road. Exercise is my way of trying to hold off any more symptoms that could surface.

My theory is if I get the body moving, challenging myself, perhaps I can slow any progression of this disorder. It scares me that it could progress.

When I look at the symptoms of MSA I have several; but they overlap with PAF. Most forms of dysautonomia have symptom overlap.

I am keenly aware that my youngest son is 12, the age I was when my dad died. And I want to be around to continue helping him grow. I know I have little control over much in life but am hopeful that working on the physical, spiritual and emotional self will produce a longer lifespan. At the least I will be calmer and happier as I go about living.

I am hopeful my diagnoses won't change. In the meantime, I am biking three to four times a week. Any more than that and I physically crash. Once the bike is hung up for winter I will swim indoors. I believe that trying to stay as healthy as possible will help.

Regardless of the outcome, biking and swimming energize me and make me feel stronger. Strong is something we don't always experience while living with a chronic condition.

PHOTOGRAPHS SHOW SMALL GLIMPSES OF LIFE

I have been taking photographs for more than 30 years. There are candids, landscapes, portraits, action shots and others. Some are posed while others are taken spontaneously. Many include people smiling. Technology allows me to edit the photos right on the screen before digitally sharing them.

Each photograph appears to tell a story. But behind that image are memories; oftentimes there is much more to the story than what the naked eye views. For the photographer sees more than the person who enjoys the final print.

Like life, what's first observed is not always the entire

story. There often are layers to a life; a story; an event; a person; or relationship.

A photograph is a snapshot in time; a moment caught; a frozen second. It may evoke laughter, happiness, joy or perhaps sadness, confusion and sorrow.

Photographs are taken for so many occasions; used to capture those moments in time. But really, they are just a small glimpse at a moment. They do not provide the smell, sounds, emotions and events that swirl around the day.

Yet, like music, a photograph can jog our memory and help recreate a moment, perhaps when we were happier, healthier or younger.

I glance at photographs and often think of before and after; the before dysautonomia and the after. It is bittersweet as I see a healthier, more energetic woman in the pre-illness photos. I was able to do so much for those first 45 years of life. And then the after photos; some of the infamous blank stare, in which I had been standing for too long and could not focus. But there are the triumphant photos, too. There is our trip to Florida, my 10-mile charity bike ride and others. And the after photographs have a common thread; I am enjoying the moment, regardless of how I feel.

Yes, photographs are not just pictures of people or an event. There is much more behind the lens.

LAST HEALTHY IMAGE CAPTURED AT WEDDING

Photographs, like music, produce feelings including excitement, fear, happiness and love.

I have a photograph of my husband and I at our niece's wedding. In it we appear happy and loving. But there is a back story. If you look closely, you can see sweat on our faces - particularly my red face - as we are in a sweltering banquet room. It is our niece's wedding reception, July 24, 2010, and we literally missed a tornado that landed less than a half mile from the hotel in which we were celebrating. Thankfully while the bridal party and nearly 200 guests drove from the wedding about 30 minutes away to the reception, no one was injured by the tornadoes that swept the area. It was frightening to see a huge tornado heading our way over the lake. We barely entered the hotel before the power went out and a twister landed down the road.

When this photograph was snapped, we were hot and tired. The reception proceeded but there were no lights, only candles. Unfortunately, the air conditioning was off, and as the evening progressed it became warmer in the banquet hall. We forgot to dance; as we were managing our three kids, seven, 12 and 17. One threw up from the heat; one was acting like a typical teen exploring a dark hotel and one was a bit fearful of the situation. We pondered whether to pack up and drive the 90-minute ride home, in the rainstorms, or stay in a sweltering, dark hotel overnight. Thankfully when we were about to leave, the electricity was restored, and we stayed the night.

There is more to this photo, much more. This photograph is the last one in which I am healthy; before chronic illness entered my life. There were tiny inklings that something was amiss, but nothing compared to what would happen a few months later and change my entire world, our world.

When I glance at this photograph, I am reminded of a heathier me. I was the person who took a long walk the morning of the wedding. I did not need a nap, and was not worried about pacing; hell I did not even know the meaning of pacing.

I could walk two to three miles back then at a fast clip, stay upright, eat whatever I wanted, drink, dance and have fun. I had no idea there was even an autonomic nervous system in our bodies let alone know it could stop working properly.

It was a different and easier time. There is no scar in the picture where my pacemaker sits; no blank stare in my eyes when I stand too long and get that look. This is a picture of the old me; the healthy me before my body failed and life as I knew it changed.

I have learned so much since this photograph was taken. I learned I have no control over much in life; some events occur and there are no good explanations of why. I've learned to rely more heavily on my faith. Relationships /people are so important, and family is crucial. And there are two choices when a body revolts; to wallow in self-pity or to continue on and do the best we can to face the new challenges.

At times, I would like to tear this photograph into tiny pieces and throw it away. But I won't. Because every moment in life gets us to the next. Every situation teaches, stretches and challenges us. It is part of this journey; called life.

I SOMETIMES FEEL LIKE A SCIENTIFIC EXPERIMENT

As I wean off a medicine that my doctor and I believe created some awful symptoms I am reminded why I began this medication more than four years ago; for migraines.

I am down to two 25 milligram pills in the morning and one in the evening. It will take at least another four to six weeks to wean completely off the medication. In the meantime, my doctor and I will meet and decide what our plan is to tackle the migraines and discern if the symptoms I am experiencing are from medication withdrawn or autonomic dysfunction.

The positives since reducing the medication are I can feel my tongue again after having had it feel numb for a long time. No doctor connected the dots that this symptom was from medication.

My heartbeat has also settled down a bit; unlike when the medication was upped, and my heart rate became more erratic; faster. My breathing and mood have improved, which is a relief.

My hands and feet feel more numb. When I sit too long the pins and needles feeling goes up my legs further than usual. I also have increased muscle/ joint pain, especially in the arms. But the worse symptom is no surprise at all, headaches. There have been at least one ocular migraine weekly since the titration began and the daily headaches are stronger.

Light and noise sensitivity is worsening. This sensitivity is what originally brought me to a neurologist in 2010 before we knew the migraines were part of autonomic dysfunction. While the medication helped with migraines, after upping the dose the side effects left me feeling unwell physically and emotionally. I decided to discontinue the medication with my doctor's approval.

My new, or perhaps resurfaced symptoms, need to be addressed when I see the doctor next month. But we agreed to get this drug out of my system before deciding our course of treatment. We need to know if there is just a migraine component or a neuropathy factor to address. Either way I feel a bit like a scientific experiment.

It is not easy to discontinue a medication after relying on it for so long. And I am reminded of two things:

1. Our bodies are complex; medical treatments need to be tweaked.
2. When there are medication changes, keep a keen eye out for physical and emotional changes, even if the medication is routine.

Chronic illness is difficult to live with; there is a lot to understand between the diagnosis and the treatment. We cannot become complacent with either or mistakes occur. I decided I was through with this medicine; the side effects of a higher dose were not worth the risks. This has caused hardships but hopefully a solution will be discerned. In the meantime, I will try to do what is best for me.

FAITH HELPS WITH CHRONIC ILLNESS STRESS

As I sit writing on Holy Saturday, Christians prepare for Easter Sunday; the beautiful day in which we commemorate the resurrection of Jesus Christ.

The church will be adorned with colorful spring flowers, banners will hang proclaiming rejoice and alleluia and for the first time since Lent began on Ash Wednesday, we will say Alleluia. Alleluia - God be praised. "He is risen! Alleluia!"

For more than 40 days Christians have been asked to reflect on the great sacrifices that Jesus made as He walked this Earth; died and rose to provide everlasting life in Heaven.

This has been the most profound Lent I can remember. I have prayed, participated in mass, reflected and attended church events but more so have realized how necessary God is in my life.

I find no coincidence in having made two trips to my Toledo cardiologist's office on Ash Wednesday and Good Friday. The first seemed routine; have the pacemaker checked/ tweaked a bit and change a medication dosage. No big deal. The second more immediate. What I discovered in looking back is that I needed God more on this journey than I knew, and having a pacemaker adds vulnerability to life.

After four weeks of feeling poorly, I tried to get my pacer settings changed; finally did; realized the local technician was inept two weeks later and traveled back to Toledo on Good Friday to see a competent technician.

I have learned a few things from this experience:

Despite my best efforts, this medical frustration left me depressed. And while having a pacemaker inside me is wonderful, because it gives me extra beats, it is really scary to think people can program my heart. They can make mistakes, or say they did one thing and do something opposite. I am now thankful I have a competent technician with Harry in Toledo, despite the 600-mile drive.

I turned away from God at the most critical point when I needed Him most. I knew I needed Him but could not pray or ask for help. And it was because I was ashamed of thoughts of not caring if I lived or died. I was sick of trying to fight day in and day out to feel somewhat ok. This went against every grain in my body, denying God and not seeking His help (sort of like Peter denied Jesus three times). I did not feel worthy of His love but knew He would give it and did give it even when I could not ask. *If you experience suicidal ideation, seek help immediately. National suicide and crisis lifeline is 988.

I hate dysautonomia. I hate what it does to me. While I try each day to do things to feel good, be productive, love and help others, sometimes the sadness, frustration, anger and loneliness grabs ahold and won't let go.

I look at people who can stand freely and really envy them, because it is such an easy act but I can't do it and am reminded of this daily. I hate sitting through church services, having to always find a place for my feet and planning out things; but I do this to survive. I don't let people know this because there is no point. And most of the time I don't give it much thought. But this Lent when I felt poorly for so long it all came crashing down on me.

I miss freedom so much. I love bike riding for many reasons, but one is because it gives me that little taste of freedom in which my legs can take me somewhere; with the wind blowing on me and the beautiful blue sky above. I long to be able to get in the car and go where I want. I must plan and cannot travel further than 45 minutes one way. This is stifling as is so much about dysautonomia.

I hate napping when my family is doing things. I feel like I am holding them back and missing out on life. When my body stops there is nothing I can do about it.

I have turned back to God. And my pastor explained that even when I thought I turned away I did not deny Him rather I was not praying, seeking Him. At those times He was carrying me, which is a very comforting belief.

What I do know is I could not continue this journey without faith. And for that I am grateful. This journey is more difficult than I often admit, and Lent reminded me of that and how much energy it takes to continue.

TIPS FOR DISCUSSING DEATH WITH LOVED ONES

Death is a difficult topic to discuss but is often helpful. Here are a few tips for talking with loved ones.

- Get a brightly colored folder. Mark it IMPORTANT. Keep it inside a fire-safe file system. Put all your pertinent documents in it including the ones noted below. Tell one person where it is located.

- Complete a Health Care Power of Attorney. Each state has a form you can complete.
- Complete a Living Will Declaration. A notary public verifies that you have signed each document.
- Talk with your adult family members about your wishes. This is a difficult topic to broach. Expect some resistance. Reflect on recent loss of life experiences. Start simple. For example, it is easier to talk about flower and music choices than burial arrangements. Start sentences with, "I prefer…"
- Make a will.
- If you hear someone say they really like something of yours, put a little sticker underneath with their name.
- These tasks are not morbid. They are gifts you are actually giving your family.
- Remember to get in photographs that are being taken. Don't let pride of how you look get in the way. Loved ones will treasure these photographs.
- Humor and jokes are normal when this subject comes up. Do the planning a little at a time; but set a deadline, no pun intended, so that you are not 'stewing over it.' When you are done with the paperwork, put it away, phew, done.
- Have a list of your bank accounts, passwords and other assets and tell someone you trust where you keep this information.

DIARY QUESTIONS

What feelings do you remember having initially after your health decline?

What feelings are you currently dealing with?

What fears do you have because of your chronic illness and how do you handle those fears?

Have you written a will or done other preplanning to let your loved one's know your plans when you die?

Chapter five: Feelings

"No one can make you feel inferior without your consent."
—Eleanor Roosevelt

"Hope is the thing with feathers that perches in the soul, and sings the tunes without the words, and never stops at all."
—Emily Dickinson

"Fear secretes acids; but love and trust are sweet juices."
—Henry Ward Beecher

Life experiences generally produce many emotions. Living with a chronic condition seems to magnify this fact. At the beginning of this journey, it is normal to feel anger, confusion, sadness, loneliness and grief. As we progress, however, we will find ways to continue to live and find happiness. This is not always an easy task and setbacks occur. Remember it is important to acknowledge feelings and seek help when necessary.

HOPELESSNESS RESULTS IN MASSIVE MELTDOWN

I crumbled to the floor and cried. I felt hopeless, frustrated and discouraged. I didn't know what to do. I had had enough. I was so sick of dealing with dysautonomia and all the trouble that it caused. I wrapped myself in a ball on the floor. I cried so hard that snot dripped out of my nose and lungs got tight.

I was crying a good 10 minutes and then I thought, what in the world am I going to do? I was so sick of this disorder. I began a new hormone replacement therapy two months earlier and thus far I feel a bit more stamina but every time I take the medicine my stomach hurts and headaches worsen. I get those horrible headaches that I can only describe as feeling like my head was put into a vice and squeezed. They are not daily but more often than I would like. I feel stuck because my Cleveland, Ohio neurologist (who was 400-miles roundtrip) moved to Wisconsin. I have an appointment with a new doctor soon. I can see my primary doctor, who is great, but he often follows the neurologist's plan. I'm unsure what to do so today I decided to lie on the bedroom floor and cry. I feel stuck, alone and scared.

Then I decided I better do something else and began to pray. The most amazing thing happened; my youngest son came bouncing in the bedroom looking for me. He lay down next to me like it was normal to find his mother on the floor. He asked me what I was doing, and I said just hanging out for a little while. He hugged me and snuggled, and we began talking about hockey. I pretended I hadn't been crying, although I'm sure he knew, and he decided the floor was comfortable. Eventually we went our separate ways; he to play and me to peddle on a stationary bike. Exercise is something I try to do to get my legs moving and to improve emotional and physical health.

My son broke up the negative thought process. He reminded me that I must continue on this medical journey. He is one of the biggest reasons I get up every morning and persevere even if life at times can depress.

ANGER, FRUSTRATION AND SADNESS RISE TO SURFACE

Three years since being diagnosed with dysautonomia and the anger, frustration and sadness grabbed me by the throat and wouldn't let go. I thought I was over that, had processed all the grief and had put it behind me. After all, I was a counselor for 23 years. I knew how to deal with feelings, right?

Recently I was surprised at the guttural reaction I had to talking about an upcoming stressful event. I thought I was anxious about the actual situation. But what surprised me even more was the flood of emotions that came pouring out about my diagnosis. I need my body to work as our daughter is having her second knee surgery in the span of 13 months. I know the drill; we arrive at the hospital at 6 a.m. and check in with the security guards; then admissions. We head up to another floor where we will check in once again. There is a lot of walking, sitting, standing and waiting. These are all things that challenge a body that is damaged by dysautonomia.

Then there is the consult with the surgeon and anesthesiologist and off to surgery for our daughter as we find a place in the waiting room with all the other relatives of loved one's having surgery. The wait could be anywhere from three to four hours at which time the surgeon will come in and report the surgery success, show pictures and give directives. Shortly afterward we walk to recovery, see our daughter and then wait. We will eventually go to a different floor and room until she wakes completely, gets dressed and then more waiting until she is released. All totaled, the day will begin around 4:45 a.m. and we will probably arrive home12-14 hours later. This is a long day for anyone, but particularly for one whose autonomic nervous system is flawed.

I realized today this all makes me angry, frustrated and sad. I long for the day when I don't have to plan how I am going to get through such an event. I want to be able to stand without becoming foggy, without feeling my heartbeat in my chest and have blood pressure either drop or rise. I long for the days when I don't have to receive a five-hour intravenous of saline the day before a big event in hopes that it keeps vital signs stable and wards off symptoms.

I long for a body that does not take so much effort just to get showered, dressed, take medications, drink fluids and get to the hospital without feeling sick. I am sure I will be one of the youngest people in the hospital wearing compression stockings and a sweater in the heat of summer. Because of the air conditioning and the length of day

I will be there, I need to do everything in my power to survive. I am fortunate to have a loving, supportive husband who knows when symptoms are getting the best of me. I will talk louder and will not be able to filter out lights and sounds. My husband will help me wait, and this is comforting. I will make it through the day; but I just wish it was not so difficult.

What I learned is that while I have handled my diagnosis well and have come to accept the limitations that have come with it, sometimes things creep up and negative feelings surface. And this is ok. This is a journey; a life-long journey with dysautonomia. I have no choice but to accept it and learn to live the best I can. What I need to remember is it is ok to have bursts of anger and sadness, they are normal, and I must acknowledge the feelings. It is important to talk about the stressors when they surface. This is part of grieving and growth.

WISHING I COULD RUN AWAY FROM LIFE FOR A BIT

I often refer to chronic illness as a roller coaster ride as there are ups and downs. I guess life in general is like that. Times are good, other times difficult. Do we persevere or give up? Some days I would like to quit this existence - run away to another land. As one of my favorite U2 songs goes:

"I want to run, I want to hide
I want to tear down the walls that hold me inside
I want to reach out and touch the flame
Where the streets have no name

I want to feel sunlight on my face
I see the dust cloud disappear without a trace
I want to take shelter from the poison rain.
Where the streets have no name, where the streets have
no name."
(Where the Streets Have No Name)

I am not sure where I would go but know that in the new existence I would be healthy and problem-free for a time. I would allow moments to relax, reflect and renew body and spirit.

The day-to-day struggles of chronic illness can become daunting at times: swallowing 28 pills and vitamins; chugging more than 120 ounces of Gatorade Zero and water; making sure to rest when needed; eating small meals; wearing compression stockings; getting weekly fluids; exercising even when feeling not up to par; planning out events to hopefully have the energy to participate; trying to keep body temperature normal. Add to this the stressors of raising a family and life can become overwhelming at times.

Chronic illness is part of life and escaping in any form only makes problems multiply.

I find comfort in this verse:

And we rejoice in the hope of the glory of God. Not only so but we rejoice in our sufferings. We know that suffering produces perseverance, perseverance character and character, hope. And hope does not disappoint us because God has poured His love into our hearts by the Holy Spirit, whom He has given us. (Romans 5:2-5)

STRESSORS OF ILLNESS CAUSE FEAR TO SURFACE

I spent most of today frightened. After beginning treatment yesterday for a sinus infection, I didn't feel well last night or today. I've been hot and cold; my blood pressure is labile; I have been nauseous; had weird dreams that I've woken from feeling like I'm going to throw up or pass out; and I feel weak and wobbly.

The worse event occurred last night. Slowly I became warm. Suddenly, I was burning hot; I thought my temperature had to be at least 103 degrees. It felt like sweat was dripping off my forehead, but it wasn't. Rather I had a body temperature of 97.7; my face was clammy and white, with blotches of red; and I asked my husband with a voice of urgency to get a cold cloth. I lay down prone on the couch for about 10 minutes until I could stand. I crawled in bed and about 20 minutes later was freezing again. The entire episode took about 40 minutes and then I curled up with three blankets and fell asleep.

It wasn't until today while replaying the scene that I realized a few things. The episode came on very quickly with little warning. I did become warm, but my temperature was bouncing from cold to warm all day. I felt sick while at the doctor's office, but I never expected to get hot so quickly. I was surprised at the intensity of the heat I experienced; then I realized when I had felt this before. While completing the Tilt Table Test (TTT) I became burning hot, this hot. Oh my goodness, I realized, I felt this nauseous and hot right before I passed out on the TTT. That is how I felt yesterday. And that is what the TTT technician warned me about; if I ever felt that way, get down, and elevate legs immediately. I was lucky I didn't pass out this time. But is this what I have to look forward to each time I am sick?

This was a simple sinus infection; I get them every fall. They seem to occur due to allergies that I have dealt with since childhood. Never have they affected me like this. So today I'm a bit angry that dysautonomia has added a new dimension to life; I'm guessing any illness will cause reactions. In addition to taking antibiotics and decongestants to recover, I must understand my body will react to the wear and tear of infection.

I spent most of the day on the couch. I prayed, slept, drank fluids, took medications, talked to friend Sharon who helped me understand what was happening and asked for help from a relative with dinner. It was a crazy day but now at least I am aware that any illness may cause added stressors.

CHOOSING HAPPINESS IS A DECISION I HAVE MADE

Being happy is a decision I deliberately make. I choose Tigger, not Eeyore. Having a damaged autonomic system is ludicrous; it's a bad joke, a dirty trick. I had an incredulous doctor once tell me that I would be dead if my autonomic system did not work. Never saw him again: "I'll show you I'm not dead!"

Wait a minute, I have stuff I must do. I resolved not to let this disorder cancel fun. I learned more about neurology, endocrinology, and hematology than I ever understood in nursing school.

I have developed a sense of humor elevated to extraordinary. It is finely tuned. I have irony because I deal with situations that would shake 'normals' to their core.

I try not to complain about minutiae. When I was in intensive care, two patients coded and did not survive. I promised God that if He let me go home, I would give up complaining (like I could give God something He needs). It was not exactly a good bargaining position, but I did return home. Not complaining liberates me.

It is almost as if I know a secret, and it makes me smile. Every now and then, from inside, a spontaneous giggle leaps out. It is a giggle much like a child watching cartoons. The small problems people fuss about do not really matter. We have lost so much yet gained insight.

I choose happy, silly, joy-filled delight. SAR

STRENGTH GROWS WHEN CHALLENGED, DESPITE FEAR

"You gain strength, courage and confidence by every experience in which you really stop to look fear in the face. You are able to say to yourself, 'I have lived through this horror. I can take the next thing that comes along.' You must do the thing you think you cannot do."
—*Eleanor Roosevelt*

I came across this quote and it resonated with me. I have found that fear is part of life; not to be relished necessarily but a part, nonetheless. We cannot sidestep nor ignore it for if we do fear germinates. Rather, we must look fear square in the eye and face its cause.

Sometimes it is difficult to know exactly where the fear comes from, other times it is evident. Evident fear for me are snakes, live or illustrated. More elusive fear is losing control.

I have learned to relinquish much control since living with dysautonomia. Before illness I was always in control. I was the person who drove everywhere, went from one place to the next nonstop and made plans far in advance. Control the environment and life went smoothly, so I thought.

All that changed when my body stopped operating efficiently and I could no longer do simple tasks like working an eight-hour day; standing in a line; driving more than 10 minutes; walking more than a 100 feet or so and standing still without becoming lightheaded. Control flew out the window and fear erupted.

As Eleanor Roosevelt so eloquently said, fear fosters confidence, courage and strength. When I notice my body revolting, instead of becoming fearful, I dive to the floor, elevate feet and drink Gatorade Zero. I am confident I can regulate my body through these accommodations. It is an automatic response to deal with stressors.

Control is gone at these moments, as there is no control when one's autonomic nervous system can go haywire without warning. In its place is confidence and strength. There is a spiritual strength, a knowledge that God walks this journey with me along with others who share the diagnosis.

Sure, fear seeps in occasionally, but mostly it is related to relationships. Will I live long enough to raise my kids? Will this illness negatively affect my family? Am I harming my kids because they live with a mom who has an illness and can't do everything they want to do? These are the fears. Mostly, however, the lack of control fosters strength in its own right.

LIFE CAN BE EXHAUSTING WHEN BODY REVOLTS

I am tired: tired of planning, preparing and pacing. Most days I must make sure to take many precautions in hopes of having a good day. Sometimes, regardless of the effort, the day is rough.

Today is a difficult day as pain is everywhere. Pain starts in my neck and shoots through the shoulders, slides down the arms to my fingertips, back and legs. My legs feel like they are being squeezed yet they have that jumpy sensation, as if I tried to rest they would not cooperate. I am guessing a combination of too much activity and four hours of sleep are the culprit for today's rough times. Coupled with the fact my heartbeat is more erratic and the calendar is filled with different appointments leading up to school for the kids, makes life feel harried.

My daughter's emotions go from happy to frustrated to angry as she tries to grasp the realities of another knee problem. I try to pretend everything will be ok, while gently preparing her in case another ACL tear or surgery occurs.

Throw this all on top of a chronic illness; trying to get a 19-year-old to realize an associate's degree in college is manageable and he can in fact achieve this goal; getting the youngest to believe he is ready for school; helping one friend as her father dies of cancer and dealing with my own feelings about this wonderful man; and having two friends newly diagnosed with illness. One a dear friend of 25 years diagnosed with Parkinson's and the other, a friend since high school, dealing with cognitive deficits since having an automobile accident.

But today I am tired. I am tired of trying to manage my Gatorade Zero intake. Tired of taking medication; small meals; having my stomach explode; not feeling normal for a consecutive period of time on any given day; tired of sitting oddly; planning what I can do; resting between activities; getting IVs; tired of it all.

Tired of not being a mom who can just do activities without exhaustion, both physical and mental. Tired, angry, frustrated, lonely, sad. Tomorrow will be better but for today I am tired of being the only one in the house up until 3:30 a.m. knowing full well this will cause hardships for the rest of the day

Tired that I am holding my family back. Just tired.

FEELING USELESS IS A HORRIBLE EXPERIENCE

The recent winter blast that left seven feet of snow on our area made something abundantly clear. My body is not capable of outdoor work. This makes me feel useless.

December reminds me of that day when I woke from an overnight sleep study, went home and proceeded to have the worse flu I can recall. I also suffered through three weeks of what I thought were migraines and vertigo and on 12/26 had no strength to get off the couch. I barely made it out of the bathtub, as my limbs felt like lead. This was my first experience with dehydration and the beginning of a spiral into dysautonomia.

Several years later, functioning is improved. However, there are moments, like when I'm stuck in the house while my family shoveled for hours, that remind me of the immense losses of this disorder.

I wonder how I can live with this forever, because forever really seems too long. Some days are long, take too much energy and I accomplish little. And then this song catches my ear. I guess God is trying to tell me something.

"BEGIN AGAIN" BY JASON GREY

"This one goes out to you
If you gave all you had and it wasn't enough
It goes out to you
If you're afraid you've failed everybody you've loved
It goes out to you
If the ties that bind are coming undone
And you're so tired that you wanna give up

189

There's never been a night so long…
There's never been a life too far gone
When you come to the end, you can begin again

It's never too late for a new start
If you give God the pieces of your broken heart
When you come to the end, you can begin again."

I don't want to give up; I am reminded that chronic means long term and right now that is daunting. I am not as physically strong as I would like, my body fails too much and there are uncertainties. Most days I get up and try to have a better day than the previous one. But I wondered this week if someday I won't care: if I will say this is enough, I am too tired to try.

How, I wonder, do we keep a realistic yet positive attitude while living with a chronic condition?

"No matter how your life's been torn apart
When you're at the end, you can begin again
There's never been a night so long…
There's never been a life too far gone
When you come to the end, you can begin again
It's never too late for a new start
If you give God the pieces of your broken heart
When you come to the end, you can begin again.
Oh, when you come to an end you got to begin again."

I continue on this journey, trust in God and see what happens.

HAVE YOU EVER WONDERED IF LIFE IS WORTH LIVING?

They say if you have enough faith in God you should not have fear. Yet when questioned of my fear I did not see it at first but then realized what exactly scared me; where it came from. I also realized while I have prayed and found some solace in knowledge that God is with me on this journey, I also pushed Him away. I did not seek Him at my darkest hour when I knew I could.

Today I went to church and prayed afterwards, thanking God for helping me see the fear; putting people in my life who care and assist.

I prayed that fear subsides along with sadness, frustration and loss of hope. The fear is not fear of death or lack of care. Rather it is fear of despair/desperation. It is the fear that I will slip into the metaphoric dark sea and not come out. I always say without hope there is not life and I believe with even a sliver of hope I will be okay. My sliver was dwindling this week and it scared me. It was a feeling I am not accustomed to experiencing.

I have wondered if chronic illness will eventually take over and I will lose all hope. Or if my body will deteriorate to that point someday. I try not to judge people on their journeys as we don't know what they deal with daily. Bodies that don't perform as we were accustomed to are difficult to handle at times.

This week brought that reality to the forefront. Between

a pacemaker not working properly and the emotions that came with it, it was perhaps the worse week I have had since this journey began. I try not to get ahead of myself but this week made things very challenging. I thought it might be easier to be dead.

And that was scary.

So, I wrote. I shared the writing with my husband, which helped me feel less alone. And I prayed, talked to my counselor and slept.

I picked the kids up from school and did what I normally do. But the sadness was palatable, and I hated it.

Three days removed I feel a bit better. But I am not back to a baseline. Today begins spring and I think the weather changing will help. And biking. And praying. And music. And writing. And reading. And telling a friend. And taking each day as it comes. And working to get my marriage on a better track. National suicide crisis lifeline is now 988.

I'M TIRED OF DEALING WITH CHRONIC ILLNESS

Sometimes my body revolts and all I can focus on is the neurological condition that took over a healthy existence. On these days my head feels like it may explode. I am dizzy, heartbeat is slow (although it can't go below 60 now that I have a pacemaker), breathing feels labored, nausea is constant, I have diarrhea and am exhausted. My blood pressure may go too low or high, sometimes I check, oftentimes not.

A friend told me early on in this journey that I would

think less and less of my chronic condition. On days like this, however, it is difficult to think of anything else.

If I could I would scream at the illness and tell it to get the hell out of my life. But there is no point to that action. Instead, I chug fluids, take extra medications to manage the additional symptoms and pain and wonder what has happened to produce these added problems? (note my doctor has allowed me to titrate or add/subtract certain medications as needed)

It is times like these in which frustration grows and the reality that this is a life-long illness hits me square in the face. Most of the time I can ignore the finality of the diagnosis or at least accept it. But when my body hurts from head to toe and the mere act of walking can be dangerous, life feels overwhelming.

I cling to hope, but the hope dwindles when the symptoms are heightened. I start questioning how I will be able to accomplish my goals. I can usually persevere but when I am flattened it is difficult.

During my most recent crash, I spent five days unable to do much more than go from one couch to the next. Finally, I got out of the house only to find myself with a stomach and head that revolted within an hour, sending me back home before finishing errands. This left me angered and frustrated. I guess furious is too strong of a word, perhaps defeated would be a better descriptor.

I was emotionally tired and sick of having plans stopped by this illness on a whim.

Sick of my life changing in an instant.

Sick of daily headaches, pain, diarrhea, brain fog and restrictions.

Sick of medicines, Gatorade Zero, no appetite and missing daily things that others take for granted like walking, standing, working, long showers, baths and eating out.

Sick of it all.
For now.
Angry.
Mad
Sad.
Defeated.
Lost.
Lonely.
Sick of it all.
Today.

TIPS FOR DEALING WITH VARIED FEELINGS

Chronic illness of any form causes challenges physically and emotionally. It is best to identify coping strategies to deal with these varied emotions. These may include:

- Find activities that utilize your strengths and produce joy. Schedule time for these activities.

- Pray.

- Research your condition but don't be obsessed with everything medical.

- Join a Facebook group tailored to your needs. Remember there will be all sorts of people with differing views and conditions. Be careful with whom you trust.

- Seek counseling if you think it would be helpful. A counselor who has worked with those with chronic illness may be an option. Make sure the counselor is qualified. Check education and credentials. Make sure they have a master's degree or above in such areas as mental health counseling or social work.

- Breathe, relax, meditate, carve time to take care of you.

- Talk to close friends whom you have identified. However, remember they have their own feelings about your situation so might not be able to understand/ help all the time.

- If you become depressed, seek help from a doctor or therapist. Sometimes depression is a result of medication or dosage changes. Depression is nothing to be ashamed of and most people experience a depressive episode at some point in their lives. It is showing strength to seek help rather than burying the emotions.

- Remember every feeling is normal. Anger, sadness, frustration, jealousy, happiness are just a few feelings we might experience. Repressing the negative feelings will not help the situation. In addition, feelings may resurface. This is the natural pattern of life.

- Look for the victories: the good in your life.

- Journal your feelings, blessings and accomplishments.

- Find things you can do.

- Count your blessings each day.

DIARY QUESTIONS

List the first five feelings that come to mind when you hear the word dysautonomia or other chronic condition?

Does your list have both feelings that are negative and positive and if so why or why not?

What strengths have you discovered in yourself since being diagnosed?

What advice would you give a newly diagnosed person?

Do you think changing our thoughts is a helpful coping mechanism?

CHAPTER SIX: RELATIONSHIPS

"I am thankful for those who said 'no.' It's because of them, I did it myself."
—*Albert Einstein*

"There is no remedy for love than to love more," Henry
—*David Thoreau*

"The only reward of virtue is virtue; the only way to have a friend is to be one."
—*Ralph Waldo Emerson*

Relationships produce both joys and sorrows. To keep a relationship strong, loved ones must learn to balance their needs with their spouse, partner, child, friend or significant other's needs. It is not an easy task. Sharon married in the middle of her spiraling health crises. I was married about 20 years when chronic illness invaded our relationship. I often speak of how the "roof" of our house had to come off a few times before my husband and I learned to communicate more effectively through crises. The roof refers to loud, long fights in which we expressed anger at one another but really were frustrated, scared and sad with the situation and our change in life's direction. It is difficult work to maintain a marriage when living with health issues. Sharon and I work at our marriages. We also think luck and the grace of God is with us.

STRENGTH NEEDED TO FIGHT THE BIG BAD WOLF

What comes to mind when I think of dysautonomia and how it changes families is the story of "The Three Little Pigs." Instead of a fragile house, this family built a strong, sturdy home, which endured all the huff and puff of the Big Bad Wolf (dysautonomia). We are a family with a home, not a house.

This story is a useful analogy to describe the buffeting of the disorder, the fragility of the structure, and the commitment by the family to make the system more secure.

Dysautonomia is not for wimps. This disorder pulls the rug out from under you. While you are in this tailspin of sorting out what is happening, family, relatives and on-lookers are wondering the same. Each goes through the stages of grief, whether it is your first-hand account of being on this roller coaster, or the bystander who can detect, sometimes before you can, that you are having an episode.

My family is astute at sensing prodrome. Take syncopal episodes seriously. Each family member absorbs the enormity of this disorder at a different pace and on a different wavelength. You can neither accelerate the process nor slow it down. If asked, make it a two-sentence teachable moment. Doubting Thomas becomes a non-voting member of parliament. He can listen but cannot vote.

"You look fine." Thank you. "You don't look sick." Gee, thanks. It's invisible. I should be awarded an Academy Award.

An acute illness is self-limiting; you drive on and recover. This Big Bad Wolf is chronic. This is difficult to fathom in a person you know to be energized, resilient, athletic and bright. I now have 16 medications prescribed. On average, adults take one medication per decade of life. At this rate, I should be 160 years old. There are times when I feel totally and utterly hideous: nauseous, flushed, hot, drenched, cold, weak, shaky, floppy upon standing, fogged, cramped and exhausted. It is neither tired, nor sleepy, nor lazy. It is beyond exhaustion. It is worse than finals' week tired; it is flattened steam-rolled tired.

Here are some suggestions of very endearing behaviors which mean the world during an episode: cover with a fleece blanket; slip your finger in one's hand; hold hair back when vomiting. This is tactile, a kind touch, which can be perceived even with low blood pressure. SAR

25 YEARS OF MARRIAGE INCLUDES TRIALS, VICTORIES

Love - it is such a small word but complex. As a nephew embarks on marriage, I ponder our own wedding 25 years ago and how marriage and love for my husband has changed.

I promise to be true to you in good times and in bad, in sickness and in health, to love and honor you all the days of my life.

On 12/30/13 my husband and I repeated our vows in

front of three dozen friends and family at the same church where we first wed. The vows held new meaning as we had history, three kids, a puppy and chronic illness in our lives.

History - the study of past events, particularly in human affairs. The whole series of past events connected with someone or something.

We've created a lot of history in our 25-year marriage and 31-years together. There has been joy and sorrow; anger and frustration; hope and despair; surprise, laughter and tears; illness and health; birth and death; success and failure.

We have seen career and job changes, three master's degrees, two apartments, three homes, many cars and vacations, three children, four broken arms, three torn ACL's and surgeries, and additional surgeries for a hernia, shoulder, gallbladder, gut, finger, arm and pacemaker.

We have attended one high school graduation, two elementary school graduations, three Baptisms and First Communions, and two Confirmations. We have buried a mother and a father. We have dealt with a chronic illness which resulted in a total change in family structure and a disability retirement at age 47. We never knew anything about the autonomic nervous system until mine decided to stop working properly three-plus years ago; now we often know more about dysautonomia than medical people we encounter.

We have attended many concerts including the Goo Goo Dolls, Billy Joel, Elton John, Sting, John Melencamp, Sarah McLaughlin, Amy Grant, Peter Gabriel, Genesis and Styx.

We have traveled to Florida too many times to count and Vermont, Toronto, North and South Carolina, Cape Cod, and now Ohio for medical reasons.

When we said our vows we had dreams. Some have been met, others modified.

We all have bicycles now and hopefully will bike as a family. I can't ride too far anymore but can go a short distance and rest; and that is alright. At least we can bike some. Families stick together despite the obstacles placed in front of them. Sometimes we must adjust our plans due to my unpredictable body, but we are learning how to navigate this road and still seize the joy that our love produces. It is not always easy and there are disappointments and sadness, but we handle it. Perhaps this is not what we envisioned on 12/30/1988 but we have had to modify our ideals.

But that is marriage, right? Learning to give and take; adjusting our expectations; changing our dreams as circumstances call. Being flexible after all is the key to life.

God changed our course; has perfect plans for us and we must trust Him.

As a 23 and 24-year-old we had no idea what we were getting into. At 48 and 49 we may have a better notion as we are more weathered. We know our plans can change in an instant. The best we can do is hold on to one another, embrace our love, trust and do the best we can in our marriage, family and life.

And the fact we still have our love is fabulous.

LEARNING TO DANCE AGAIN AS A COUPLE

I don't believe in New Year's resolutions but rather reflections. The year 2013 was interesting, challenging, sorrowful and hopeful. I am glad to put the year to rest and begin anew; hopeful that the dawning of my 50th year on this earth will be productive and full of happy surprises.

When I gaze back on 2013 there is a theme that weaves through life - dancing. I learned to dance. It was not the dancing one does with a partner when your feet go back and forth listening to music. Rather there was a beat; a life beat.

This dancing was more about learning how to navigate (dance through) difficult situations with my love. We grabbed each other as we swayed back and forth through each event we faced and worked hard not to step on each other's toes in the process.

We learned how to communicate better, deal with difficult situations and hold on tightly during each ride we encountered. We dealt with three surgeries and near death for his mom; ACL surgery and rehabilitation for our daughter and pacemaker surgery for me; along with trying to sell a home and raise three kids and a puppy. We had great things happen too - including our son graduating from high school; our first family vacation in years; and our 25th wedding anniversary which included a vow renewal and dinner party. There was much dancing in 2013.

We became better listeners to each other's needs. Instead of stepping on toes and putting individual goals first, we negotiated, read each other better and compromised.

These things get lost sometimes in the day-to-day drudgery of life; throw in chronic illness and perhaps it is one more stressor that helps one lose sight of fundamental necessities.

We dread doctor appointments together; he because there are long miles to drive and traveling seems to put the fact I have a medical condition in our immediate views. Me because he turns grumpy and stressed as he gets nearer to the appointment while I look at the visit as a means of hope; a way to change medicines, get more information, try something new and perhaps feel a bit better. But appointments tax my body and our family, despite the fact I pre-plan as much as possible. I still feel as if I burden the ones I love the most.

Things shifted, however, during a pacemaker follow-up appointment in Toledo. My husband and I went to dinner and had fun despite unappetizing food. We laughed, talked and enjoyed one another; our first time at an actual restaurant in a long time. The next day we waited three hours, between an unexpected medical test I needed and a late specialist, to see the doctor. I watched my husband tire, felt my annoyance rise. He would rush me during the appointment; I would get angry; it would be a long 300-mile ride home, I thought. I did something unexpected; I suggested he go for a walk, get lunch and unwind. He came back and still no doctor. I sent him off again, realizing I needed him out of the room so I could take all the time necessary without worrying. I suggested he go rest in the car; he was relieved to know I could stay focused during the appointment, and he could unwind. Dysautonomia robs me at times of focusing as the brain tires. My husband supports me but I knew it was time to support him. We were learning to dance again together, and it worked. He rested and was ready for a long drive home in the dark with challenging weather. And I spent as much time with my cardiologist as necessary.

I am sure there will be more challenges in our future but joy does indeed come from sorrows. But I also am convinced our dance steps will continue to align.

CHRONIC ILLNESS INTRUDES ON RELATIONSHIPS

If I had to pinpoint a common theme of this chronic illness journey, I would pick relationships.

Relationship - the way in which two or more people, groups, countries, etc., talk to, behave toward, and deal with each other. The way in which people are connected.

My relationships have flourished since a dysautonomia diagnosis. Not all of them, granted. Sadly, some people have left my life, the non-believers per se. These are the people who had a difficult time understanding how someone that looks outwardly healthy is unwell. They are the people whom either are afraid to be near me, perhaps uncomfortable with their own mortality, or aren't sure how to deal with the challenges I face. They might come around occasionally but since I can no longer do the activities I once could they see me infrequently. This saddens me but I cannot control other's actions, only my own.

The new and strengthened relationships are a true blessing, however. As a trained counselor I listened a lot in my professional life. Chronic illness has afforded me the time and will to listen more astutely to others. I'm amazed at the feelings I have when I'm in the presence of others. When I tell someone our conversation or meeting that day was a blessing, I am sincere.

This is the gift of the relationship that chronic illness and God has blessed me with.

WE ALL FEEL VULNERABLE AT TIMES

Vulnerability- susceptible to physical or emotional attack or harm. Helpless, defenseless, powerless, impotent, weak, susceptible.

I hate the vulnerability that can occur while living with chronic illness; absolutely hate it.

I was recently reminded of this when a misunderstanding occurred with a friend. My intentions were pure but she misread them and reacted in a way I hadn't expected. I had crashed physically during a meeting; my face felt hot, brain was not processing information, hands were purple, body cold. I was having a difficult time focusing on what was being said and I was sitting with legs elevated, hoping I would quickly recover.

I chugged 20 ounces of Gatorade and was about to ask my friend to get me a second bottle from the refrigerator when what I said upset her and terminated our communication for the day. It was not what I said, but lack of delivery, caused by lost social skills due to fogging, that resulted in our misunderstanding.

When I recovered enough to get home, I realized what upset me almost as much as our rift was the vulnerability I felt. I was no longer this competent, smart woman that could run a support group for those with chronic illness. No, I was a person who fights every day to live as normal a life as possible despite illness. I am aware nearly hourly of the fact I have dysautonomia and must make decisions accordingly. These decisions include whether to wear compression socks, layer clothes properly and spend limited energy. And when I make errors, my body will let me know, through headaches, dizziness, pain, digestion problems, exhaustion and more. Even when I follow the plan exactly the body may revolt. No two days seem the same.

It is difficult to live this way, let alone explain it to others. So when someone I trust reacts in a manner I am unaccustomed too, it brings out the feelings of vulnerability. And it makes me think twice before sharing the true depths of what this illness does on a daily basis.

FEELING BETRAYED BY HEALTH, LOVED ONE

Autonomous- self-directing freedom and especially moral independence. Acting independently or having the freedom to do so.

My autonomy was ripped from me. It was as if a thief came in, grabbed it and ran before I could blink, think or breathe. I was left blindsided, stunned and saddened. The worse part: the thief was my husband.

In a broader sense the thief is dysautonomia and always will be. But in this instance my husband betrayed me; stole my freedom and autonomy. This fact is difficult to admit and face. Because he is the one person, the only person, in this world who sees the day-to-day grind that chronic illness creates. He supports and loves me and I trust him. But when things like this occur, I lose a bit of trust and it is difficult.

Dysautonomia has robbed me of the freedom to do the things I want, when I want. In this case I cannot drive long distances so must rely on others to transport me to out-of-state doctor appointments. On this occasion, traffic jams and confusion caused stress in our car; coupled with increased symptoms/fogginess from sitting too long. We argued and while I spent several hours at the cardiology clinic my husband stewed, fueling his frustration at the illness.

Even though it was 7 p.m. when I rejoined him and we had already driven 300 miles that day, he decided we were going home; another 300 miles in the dark. I would not be seeing my dear friend the next day in Cleveland; a planned three-day visit.

At that very moment I was so sad, angry and alone. I was stuck in that car with nowhere to go; no way to get out. I believed I was a useless person who could not take care of myself. I was unable to drive to a cardiologist appointment or to a friend's home. I was stuck and the person I loved the most seemed to have betrayed me. I felt hopeless.

And I prayed.

After about an hour, we talked and decided to get a hotel for the night. At check-in, the clerk said the room must have been meant for us because she turned down the last person; there was one room left; and God must have had a plan for us.

We settled in and had a restful sleep. And I sit writing this from my friend's home, because the mini retreat occurred. I am thankful my husband and I worked through our differences.

We are reminded that chronic illness will always challenge our marriage. While it appears easier to pretend it does not affect us, it is a constant stressor. Medical visits remind us that I do have needs that cannot be ignored. Sometimes the pressure causes our relationship to unravel; sometimes not.

Either way we must persevere, talk, laugh, and love.

SUPPORT GROUP PROVIDES HOPE TO ALL

It's the group no one wants to join but we are all happy to have met. It is comprised of 11 women and two men, ranging in age from 40s to 70s. We talk, share, nod, listen, pray, eat and cry. We have one main thing in common: chronic illness.

We are a HopeKeepers* group I began with a friend at church. I would never have dreamt of starting such a group, but my path has taken this turn and I am excited. I had scoured the internet for hours on end and could not find any chronic illness support group in the area. There were plenty of groups for specific needs but nothing for chronic illness. I was lonely and looking for others to meet who understood the reality of a chronic condition.

I called the Catholic Diocese of Buffalo and talked with the coordinator of disability services. They say God works in mysteries ways and before I knew it I was not only volunteered to run a group, but was also the new parish advocate for the chronically ill and disabled at my church.

You would think a group for people with illnesses would be depressing but it is not. We talk about the loss and sadness, but we also have the hope that our futures will be prosperous. We all have realized we have to reinvent ourselves a bit. God gives me the endurance to sit with these inspiring men and women for two hours twice a month and listen, share and be enriched.

We are a diverse group of people from several different religious backgrounds. We share, support and listen to one another and are truly blessed.

*HopeKeepers is a group originally developed by Lisa Copen. Lisa lives with chronic illness. She began a Christian ministry to support others with the same issues. She is an author and friend.

DAILY PLANNER IS A REMINDER TO TRY TO FLOURISH

I have a daily planner. It states positive thoughts and includes pictures. It is the second yearly planner in the series I have purchased. I like it for three reasons; it is hope-filled, sturdy and reminds me to improve my attitude on days in which I am less than positive. A recent statement read something like this: if you stumble, remember where and how it feels. Tomorrow take a different path. Life flourishes from its pain and the lessons we learn.

After reading this, I wonder if some people are thinking their lives must really be flourishing if pain is the variable. After all, those with chronic conditions know a thing or two about pain; both physical and emotional. Whether it be pain in muscles and joints or the pain of lost relationships, careers, and dreams; there is plenty of pain to share.

Where is all the flourishing, thriving? As a leader of a HopeKeepers group for chronically ill people in my community, I work with those in different stages of illness. We are a group from all walks of lives, ages, socio-economic levels. We have at least two things in common - chronic illness and our belief in God.

The people in the group, like everyone, have suffered in their own ways. What I observe, however, is this. Most have a deep connection to God. They rely on Him daily for spiritual, emotional and physical strength to handle that which is put in front of them. One woman with multiple sclerosis gives an example of being stuck on the floor unable to get up. "Ok God, I need you, give me the strength in my legs to get back in my wheelchair." And He did.

We all have stories of suffering; if we pay attention, we also have victories. And to have God walk this journey with us is remarkable.

EVEN WHEN WE CAN'T GO OUT, WE NEED FRIENDS

Have you ever imagined standing up in front of friends and family and telling them the truth about how it feels to live with a chronic condition? Or fantasized about telling others about the things that you have experienced since diagnosis that have been hurtful or resulted in loneliness. Oftentimes, it is difficult to share these thoughts and if we try the audience does not always hear the message; rather becomes dismissive or defensive. Here are 16 things we would like our loved ones to understand.

We love spending time with you; but oftentimes it will result in exhaustion. Coming over to our home to watch a movie or talk may be easier than going out.

Remember we are still people, just like you. We may not be able to perform all the tasks we previously enjoyed but our spirit lives. In fact, we often have a greater appreciation for the little things, the blessings in life. Relationships are blessings.

We may forget things, repeat ourselves or get loud. Brain fog sets in, especially due to fatigue or sitting too long. Please be patient.

We get lonely. Most people around us go to work or school, while we are home alone for upwards of half the day. Sometimes we just need human conversation to feel alive.

Simple things like meeting for tea/ coffee at a local shop is wonderful. A large meal oftentimes takes too much time and causes digestive issue.

We get scared. With conditions like dysautonomia,

which is not rare but rarely diagnosed in a timely fashion, we must advocate for treatment. Many of us travel to other states from home just to see a competent doctor. This becomes frustrating. What is more frustrating and frightening, however, is when we need immediate care and there are few options in our geographical area.

It is difficult for us to ask for help. We want to remain independent, but unfortunately there are things we just cannot do anymore. If we seek assistance, we must really need some help. Try to assist if you can.

Don't think because we live with a chronic condition you should not " bother us" with your problems. This makes us feel less than important and honestly is not the way to foster relationships. We can talk, listen and be supportive of our loved ones so please remember to share your celebrations and struggles. We care.

Don't stop inviting us to events. I have teared up when I have seen photographs on social media of friends doing things together that I could easily have performed. Let me have the opportunity; if I can't do it I will say so. But keep inviting me. And please don't take it personally if I decline or cancel at the last minute. My body is unpredictable and despite best efforts it flattens me at times.

Allow us to modify our environment, rather than assisting us. I must keep my feet up, otherwise I feel like I will pass out. I either find a second chair or sit in a position that works for me. I know how to handle my condition; and while you are trying to be helpful when offering a chair or other tool, I want you to know I can handle these situations. I will ask if help is needed.

Don't feel sorry for us. Most of the time we do not feel this way. We embrace life and try to do our best each day. Pity is one of the worse aspects of this life

Don't ask us what we do all day. Sometimes days are productive and other times we might need to sleep. Either way, we listen to our bodies and try to pace activities. We cannot go from one activity to the next; our energy supply is more finite. We would love to have boundless energy, but we don't. Remember we don't ask you what you do all day on your days off; and when we hear this question presented to us, we often cringe. It also devalues us.

Treat us like you would other friends and relatives. We are people; that has not changed.

Understand that while we might look healthy on the outside all sorts of body systems inside are rebelling. We won't talk about all these things but please know we don't fake it.

Understand that we choose to have fun but oftentimes will have to pay the price later. Recovering from activities may take hours or days; but we would rather try to live/ enjoy ourselves than not.

Please know we are thankful that you are in our lives. We have lost friends and relatives. This is a fact of living with chronic illness. We are not sure why but speculate some don't believe us; some are afraid our illness is contagious; and some are fearful as they realize life can change quickly. Thank you for staying.

TIPS FOR DEALING WITH CHANGING RELATIONSHIPS

Illness in a family causes added stressors. Below are suggestions to improving communications with the one's you love.

- Be honest with each other. Don't let emotions stew and don't fail to work on issues.

- In a marriage or intimate relationship, realize there will be shifts. Negotiate, talk and remember to listen. Understand the healthy partner worries about their partner's health and the issues this creates.

- Remember that both people see the effects of dysautonomia daily. Encourage the healthy partner to still live; get out and do activities they enjoy. Have them take pictures so you can see what enjoyment is occurring.

- Share with your partner but remember you do not have to tell them every symptom. Filter a little so not to overwhelm them more.

- Look for angels - those surprise people that will come in your life or who are already present who do things to help, understand and love. Tell them how much their actions are appreciated. Remember relationships are difficult when both members are healthy and more difficult when chronic illness enters the situation. Seek professional help as needed.

DIARY QUESTIONS

How have your relationships changed since diagnosis?

Have you lost relationships?

Gained relationships? How do you nurture relationships despite feeling awful at times?

What are three things you can do to improve a relationship that is important to you?

CHAPTER SEVEN: WORDS

"He who has a why to live, can bear almost any how."
—Friedrich Nietzsche

"To love oneself is the beginning of a lifelong romance."
—Oscar Wilde

"Well done is better than well said."
—Benjamin Franklin

"When ideas fail, words come in handy."
—Johann Wolfgang von Goethe

The English language is comprised of more than one million words. Words are powerful in both the written and spoken forms. Some words produce wonderful feelings. These words may include love, faith, hope, and for me personally chocolate. Other words evoke negative thoughts and feelings. These may include death, chronic, surgery and prejudice. The following are words that may evoke feelings, whether negative or positive.

LIVE, BE WELL

I put a new bracelet on- a purple band, stone material with four simple letters that spell the word live. I wear it under my wrist so I can see the word often; a constant reminder to embrace life.

Live - to be alive.

To maintain oneself.

To have life rich in experience.

As I begin my fifth decade of life, I am reminded of how fortunate I am to be alive in this century. I have out-lived my father's age by three years and am very aware of my own mortality. But 2014 is much different than 1976 when he died prematurely despite taking very good care of himself. Circumstances beyond his control - a hor-rific firefighting accident in 1964 - began his myriad of chronic health issues beginning two months prior to my birth. Health care was not advanced enough to prevent his medical problems or save him from a massive, fatal heart attack.

Fast forward 38 years and I too am retired from my career with a disability pension. As my dad before me, I strive to live life with joy and integrity; relishing rela-tionships especially those of my children, husband, close friends and God. I am fortunate to have better health care than the previous generation and a pacemaker ticking almost nonstop inside me to give my heart the boost it needs to help me feel better. In turn, today's medicines and vitamins are more advanced than they were from 1964-76.

Dad too lived, very well, despite pain, illness and disappointment. He was my role model, and I am thankful for the 12 years he physically graced my life. He continues to influence me in spirit as a constant reminder of the amazing good there is in life.

As I turn 50, I look back on the half century in awe and bewilderment. Of course, some goals were met. I am married to the only man I have loved, have three kids and had two great careers, as a writer and school counselor. We purchased three homes; just recently one that feels like we might stay in it for a long time. We are working to raise our kids and my relationship with God has grown tremendously.

And then there was the major curveball - the illness that changed the direction of our lives; my career; our goals. What seemed like a simple aborted bike ride because I was dizzy and my heart rate was unstable turned out to be much more. This bike ride at the age of 46 turned our lives' upside down; sending me to doctor after doctor for nearly a year until dysautonomia was diagnosed.

The adventure continues but the initial crises has subsided. Now it is a matter of managing the varied symptoms that come with a faulty autonomic nervous system.

One of the most important things for me to remember is to live and embrace life; to relish the joys when they come.

I decided early on in this journey that if I am having a good hour, I try to enjoy that time. When I am with someone, I attempt to offer them full attention and embrace our time together. When I am in church, I do my best to really listen to the Gospel readings and attempt to understand what message is offered.

Fear creeps in - how will I die; will I live to see my kids grow; will this disorder progress; will I ever improve or get considerably worse? But mostly I pray, trust, embrace life and do the best I can to live.

Everyone has burdens, everyone has joys. No one truly understands what someone else experiences. The best we can do is listen, be with others and love one another.

As I enter my 50's I hope I can continue to grow and support others as I live the best life possible.

When I left my Toledo cardiologist's office, he offered me three words. I believe they sum it up. Live. Be well.

BALANCE

Balance - an even distribution of weight enabling someone or something to remain upright and steady; a condition in which different elements are equal or in the correct proportions.

Balance while living with dysautonomia is tricky at best, oftentimes impossible. Some days I stumble while standing still, as if the floor has moved. I look around, however, and few others are plagued by this condition. If I am with family, we chuckle at this sudden loss of balance.

Pre-diagnosis I was aware when floors and pathways were uneven. Others seemed unaware and I wondered why? I bought steady, firm shoes to help keep footing secure.

Our new home is 64 years old and some floors slant. We found out it was built over a former glass factory and railroad path. The ground is not as solid as we would have presumed; perhaps causing the uneven floors due to settling. Regardless, I occasionally lose footing in the home, and am cognizant of the floors' dips and dives. They are subtle, but ever present. Perhaps for someone with a healthy autonomic nervous system there is no concern, but for me I know that the terrain can cause trouble.

Balance is a key to life and living with dysautonomia brings that to the forefront. I must make choices each day to keep life in check. These choices include taking vitamins and medications on time; exercising; making sure I don't stand or sit too long; conserving energy for planned events; and drinking enough fluids to stay ahead of the constant threat of dehydration.

Balance.

I marvel at the fact I maintain enough balance to ride my Trek 24-speed hybrid bicycle. Somehow, I can keep my body upright without tipping. I am thankful for this gift. I can't ride as far as I could before dysautonomia, but I accept this new reality.

I struggle with balance as each bike ride feels marvelous but then I crash physically afterwards. Most rides are uneventful but one to three hours later I am exhausted and my body revolts. I had to stop in the middle of a recent ride, put my feet up and chug fluids as I was lightheaded. I recovered and finished but the rest of the day left me symptomatic (I wear a helmet, carry a cell phone and medic alert bracelet for safety). Now I ponder what to do to enjoy the rides and not crash so hard.

If I can't find a solution, I have decided I will accept the reality of what happens physically after biking. Because the ride - the freedom, the amazing, glorious feeling of using leg muscles to peddle again after losing that joy for more than a year- is worth it.

And I will continue to wrestle with keeping myself upright and on a steady path in this world in which I live.

HUMOR IS NECESSARY

Humor - the quality of being amusing or comic, especially as expressed in literature or speech.

I have had so many MRIs, I might stick to the refrigerator.

This book is not a pity party. Laura and I have written it in part as a guide to help the reader grasp how difficult it is to arrive at a name/diagnosis for our symptoms. We often resemble Lucy and Ethel of I Love Lucy on their various escapades.

Any time bodily fluids are involved there is opportunity for humor. We are stripped of so much but can still hang on to our funny bone. Things that we share with each other would only partially be appreciated by the well public.

Jokes that we have heard a hundred times are still funny, and even a word may make us convulse in laughter.

An example is if either of us mentions protein shake guzzled prior to a TTT, we begin to laugh and reminisce. For Laura and I, this brings back vivid memories of trying to get her safely to her TTT. She could barely walk straight because she was off medications. She insisted, however, to chug a protein shake in the hospital lobby even though I warned her against this action. During the TTT, after passing out, she nearly puked the protein shake. We still laugh about that crazy experience.

To deal with frustration or comic relief there is an assortment of marshmallow and confetti launchers. We joke about which annoying people to shoot with these toys.

We offer comradeship in this discovery. There are times you teach the teacher; steady your course, fly a high kite.

If all else fails, there is always chocolate. SAR.

SYNCOPE

Syncope - to cut short (Old Greek). The loss of consciousness due to insufficient blood flow to the brain; faint.

If found unconscious, speculation is that you are drunk, diabetic, epileptic or faint. Label yourself. Keep your medical identification or bracelet up to date.

To your own self be true. Who are you kidding? You get the warning: the oh no notion which includes clammy skin, vision and hearing changes, knees that buckle, body swaying and extremely hot or cold. Sit or lie down immediately. Elevate your legs so that they are higher than your heart. You may look strange but who really cares?

If you fall, the injury sustained could be serious. It could result in three co-morbids: faint, fall, and injury. If that happens, recovery is complex.

In an effort to avoid syncope, always take your medication and refill prescriptions on time. Stay hydrated. Avoid alcohol which dehydrates. Carry fluids always. SAR

DETOURS

Detours - roundabout or circuitous way or course, especially when used temporarily when the main route is closed; an indirect or roundabout procedure, path, etc.

I am reading a book in which the main character keeps experiencing detours while trying to reach her goal.

I can't help but think of my own life and all the detours I have encountered. I imagine all our lives have detours and we have choices; grab on and embrace the different paths our lives take or crumble.

I know some days I feel like crumbling. These days are often the ones in which my body hurts more than usual. Perhaps digestion is worse than normal, I am dizzy, light headed or am dealing with a constant headache. Whatever the cause, energy level is nonexistent regardless of what I do to feel better.

Thankfully since having a pacemaker implanted I have less of these days. I still crash (a crash is when my vital signs go so haywire that I have to lie flat, get my feet up, snuggle under a blanket and rest as anything else is too taxing) but a full day of horrible symptoms does not occur as often as it did before the pacemaker. Detours are less frequent.

The pacemaker certainly was a detour I never expected. And while at first, I did not embrace the surgery, eventually I accepted the challenge and have become accustomed to having a device. Other detours: my career ended, health declined, and I had to learn different ways in which to go about the day. I stopped taking for granted simple things including exercising daily and standing in a line as these things became impossible.

Amazing things have also occurred on my detoured life. I have met many new people; have grown in my faith; value relationships more; have opportunities to help others who are new to dysautonomia or chronic illness and spend more time with my kids and husband.

Sometimes certainly there is sadness of the old life but there has to be trust that the detour will bring about a path valuable in its own right. It may not be evident at first but with time, it becomes crystallized.

ACCEPTANCE

I have been flattened for three days, something I haven't experienced in a while. My body revolted sending me spiraling physically. Thankfully, the in-home health care agency plugged me into its schedule and with three bags of IV fluid over a two-day period I am beginning to feel more like a person, rather than a blob of inertia taking up space on the living room couch.

I even took a shower without my heart pounding so hard that I felt it would explode. I always feel a bit better with clean clothes and fresh smells. I could finally wipe the blood off my hand from the successful IV start after two misses. I was quite dehydrated, and this coupled with a nurse who didn't know my veins proved challenging in starting a line.

I haven't crashed this hard in months and it made me realize, once again, that dysautonomia is in my life until I die. And that is difficult to comprehend.

Acceptance - willingness to tolerate a difficult or unpleasant situation.

I don't think total acceptance is ever possible nor helpful when dealing with chronic conditions. I'm not advocating denial, but we need to at best hope for improvement. Staying stagnant is not beneficial. We can hold on to our fighting spirit; a willingness to work to feel better; changing up the routine; trying new medications; seeking different treatment options.

I review medications with my specialist and primary care doctor at each visit to see if anything can be tweaked to improve functioning. I also question both doctors about any research I have found- or they have- which might be of benefit.

Unfortunately, the funding for dysautonomia research is limited. So, while we are realistic and accept our diagnosis we also need to serve as advocates for treatment.

Sometimes advocating is difficult, especially when the

body revolts. This leaves us miserable, flat and unable to stand upright without serious symptoms.

It is a balancing act at times - literally. Balancing on two feet - often known as standing upright- can be a vast challenge. There is also balancing our fluid intake, medications, emotions, energy output and rest. All this can be set off balance by almost anything, from weather changes to a cold to stress. Our bodies have nervous systems that do not operate properly and despite our best efforts we get knocked off balance and end up on the couch for days, needing fluids either at home or in an emergency room.

We persevere, however, because that is in our nature.

OCCASIONAL WELLNESS

People often hear the term chronic illness. Chronic meaning long-term, constant; and illness a disease or sickness effecting the body or mind. This term may conjure up negative images of people struggling to live. But there are many people, of all ages, that embrace life despite their health.

As someone diagnosed with chronic illness, I began to ponder this term. It is negative while my life is not. Sure there are struggles, but everyone faces such. There are also gains that come from learning to do things differently because a body does not cooperate the way it once did. There are emotional and spiritual growths that I am convinced would never have occurred without a medical diagnosis.

I decided to take the words chronic and illness and find a better descriptor. Perhaps I won't be able to convince the medical field of this but my counselor training tells me that reframing- or basically changing up the way something is presented- can shift the way people view the struggle. For instance, instead of calling a child hyperactive we can call them enthusiastic or energetic; a person who never stops talking could be said to have a lot on their mind. So why not take the term chronic illness and reframe it?

The opposite of chronic is occasional.

The opposite of illness is wellness.

And there you have it; I no longer have a chronic illness rather I have occasional wellness.

Occasional- occurring, appearing, or done infrequently and irregularly.

Infrequent- intermittent, sporadic, odd, random.

Wellness- the quality or state of being in good health especially as an actively sought goal.

Healthiness- heartiness, wholeness.

And this is true; for each day there are moments, perhaps minutes, sometimes hours in which I can do things that I want or need to do with little effort. Sure there is preplanning and weighing the consequences of choices compared to the energy used. But there are occasional times in the day when I feel well; healthy; whole.

When I am riding a bicycle through the village and my heart is pounding, legs are working and I am glancing around taking in the beauty of life, I am well.

I am well at other times too; and most often I notice, because it feels remarkable. I can't say it is symptom - free but more stable, less nauseous, light-headed and such. It is an occasional wellness that I embrace. It is happier and more fulfilling than a chronic illness which sounds very depressing.

It is semantics and neither changes the fact the body does not work properly and probably never will again. But occasional sounds good to me; wellness is what I strive for. I know I have an edge in some areas over more healthy people as I savior the moments; the blessings; the relationships.

I am wholeheartedly thankful for the life I have. I am living the best I can.

SERENITY

God grant me the serenity to accept the things I cannot change, the courage to change the things I can and wisdom to know the difference.

We have heard this popular part of the Serenity Prayer by Reinhold Niebuhr. And living with chronic illness there is so much we cannot change. I cannot change the circumstances of my illness or the fact it at times wreaks havoc on my family life

But: I can change my attitude about how I look at these situations. I can remember that despite disappointments, worries and losses, God is always on this journey. In fact God is way ahead. If life looks bleak, or makes no sense, there is still a plan that God has put in motion. Oftentimes we have no idea what the plan is for weeks, months, even years. But there is always a plan. Always.

It is difficult to decipher what is changeable and what cannot change. There is much in our lives we have no control over, and that is where faith comes in. We must rely on God at all times but faith is also critical when we are in our darkest moments.

Here is the beautiful conclusion of the Serenity Prayer.

Living one day at a time;
Enjoying one moment at a time;
Accepting hardships as the pathway to peace;
Taking, as He did, this sinful world
As it is, not as I would have it;
Trusting that He will make all things right
If I surrender to His Will;
So that I may be reasonably happy in this life
And supremely happy with Him
forever in the next.
-The Serenity Prayer by Reinhold Niebuhr

ROCKS PROVIDE COMFORT TO GROUP MEMBERS

I brought a dozen rocks to a HopeKeepers meeting. Each rock had a word inscribed; hope, blessed, believe, trust, strength, pray and others.

After we said a prayer asking the Holy Spirit for guidance, each member randomly chose a rock. What happened next was remarkable. Each member stated that the exact word received was something they needed. One woman revealed pray on her rock.

"I have gotten away from daily prayer and just began to

focus more on it, " she said. "This rock is a good reminder."

Another person stated that her blessed stone reminded her of the constant struggle she was having with identifying blessings while dealing with several illnesses.

I didn't look at my rock until it was my turn to talk. When I glanced at the word I was awestruck.

Believe - to have firm religious faith; to accept something as true, genuine or real; to have a firm conviction as to the goodness, efficacy, or ability of something.

I knew my rock was God inspired. I was having a difficult time trusting God. Several things had happened, and I was floundering. I still prayed, attended church; but something was missing.

And God once again was reminding me to believe and trust.

That belief was challenged when I sat at my beloved mother-in-law's bedside. She survived surgery to repair a blown aneurysm but the effects were irreversible; she died three days later. I had my believe rock with me, as I always do. I prayed aloud in her room; prayers that I've known since childhood. They were of comfort to me and I believe she could hear me.

We are constantly challenged with our health issues. It is easy to give in to the negative thoughts; stop believing. But I am convinced these rocks are just one more affirmation that we must hold on to hope and faith.

GOD OVERRULES SURGEON IN MEDICAL PROCEDURE

"Keep looking," I said to the orthopedic surgeon after he stated he could not find a two-centimeter tear in the rotator cuff while operating on my left shoulder early that July morning.

I was dazed from medication but alert enough to know I wanted him to make sure he didn't miss anything while inside my shoulder. I knew not to speak to the doctor unless spoken to and he had just told me he could not locate the tear, despite seeing it in his office four months earlier on a magnetic resonance imaging (MRI).

The block given to me during surgery did not reach the entire area and I felt slight twinges during the operation. I did not care, however, as I was more concerned that the surgeon did a thorough job.

The doctor cleaned bone fragments, bursitis and other "junk" out of my shoulder as I watched on a computer monitor. It was fascinated to observe this man's skill; to see the inside of the human body, what God has created, was indescribable. But the surgery ended there, as there was no tear.

I went home thankful surgery was over and my autonomic nervous system tolerated it. But more dramatic was the fact that my rotator cuff was intact, and my recovery would be far less extensive. Instead of being immobilized for months I would be in a sling for just a week and start physical therapy two weeks later. Now two months out I have pain, but I am gaining mobility and the recovery will not take the expected year.

Miracle - a surprising and welcome event that is not explicable by natural or scientific laws and is therefore considered to be the work of a divine agency.

The day after surgery was my birthday. Forty-eight years earlier I was born prematurely, and my dad had come home and told my siblings I was not expected to live, rather I would go to Heaven. My family refers to it as a miracle that I survived. I believe my second miracle came when the surgeon could not find that tear in my shoulder _ the one visible on the MRI.

I told my primary care physician and the nurse practitioner who participated in the surgery my theory during follow-up appointments. Neither could explain medically what happened and both agreed that yes indeed I just may have gotten a miracle.

So I rejoice in the fact that while I'm living with a chronic illness God cut me a break that day in the operating room and I am forever grateful.

WAITING FOR DOCTOR APPOINTMENT TESTS PATIENCE

Sixteen months. I waited 16 months for a doctor appointment. It was not by choice. That is how long it took to secure an appointment with one of the top specialists for dysautonomia in the country. I didn't think I would ever get to see him, but it finally occurred. After traveling 300 miles each way, I saw this world-renowned cardiologist Dr. Blair Grubb- the man who conducted volumes of research on dysautonomia.

It was a remarkable doctor's appointment. He spent more than two hours with my husband and me, answering our questions. He treated me like a person and even quoted the Bible. The doctor is a great historian, evident by many stories; a human being; a person who understands that the medical journey patients are on is not pleasant and his empathy showed through. He listened, explained and understood.

> **Patience - the capacity to accept or tolerate delay, trouble, or suffering without getting angry or upset.**

Patience is so difficult, but with chronic illness there is often no other choice. We wait for doctor's appointments; tests to be scheduled; results and then decisions. Sometimes we wait to get better, but oftentimes that does not occur.

Each time I prepare for the 600-mile journey to see this specialist, I have the knowledge that the doctor will listen and try to do his best to help me with this life-long condition. It is an act of faith and great patience. I have more questions to ask; symptoms to explore, decisions to make. I also have the knowledge that the doctor will listen and try to do his best to help me with this life-long condition. It is an act of faith and great patience.

SCARS BOTH PHYSICAL AND EMOTIONAL

> **"Scars are souvenirs you never lose, the past is never far." *Name* by the Goo Goo Dolls**

I have several scars on my body and within my heart.

Scars to remind me of shoulder, gallbladder and appendix surgery. I also have "heart" scars; probably the greatest was witnessing my dad die of a massive heart attack when I was 12.

Scars - a mark left by the healing of injured tissue. A lasting emotional injury.

In nine days, I add another scar to my body - one that will touch my heart in both physical and emotional ways - when I get a pacemaker to help correct bradycardia.

The scar will be about 3.5 inches long, a constant reminder that my heart needs assistance to beat properly due to a faulty autonomic nervous system. My dad died in 1976 at the age of 48 before medical technology was advanced enough to know how to repair such problems. He did not have bradycardia, but at 49 I have outlived him and wonder if he would have had a much longer life if medicine were more advanced in his time.

My father would be pleased to know my heartbeat can be corrected with technology. This opportunity, though it scares me, hopefully will return   some of the lost energy that dysautonomia has stolen.

It frightens me to have someone tinker with heart rhythms. I am sure the vulnerability comes from my "heart scars." But I also know if I don't take this chance, I will continue to be a person with all the spirit of my old self but less than half the energy. I will be the mom that watches the kids from the sidelines. I miss event after event, whether it be a dinner out with family, a sporting or school function. When I do make it to an event, it comes with great preplanning and oftentimes a physical crash afterwards.

As my kids continue to grow, there will be more challenges: confirmations, high school and college graduations, weddings, and grandchildren. Instead of worrying about which moments I can participate in and which I will miss it would be remarkable if I could be present for everything.

The scar will be my souvenir, as will the small pacer that will help the heart beat more steadily. It will be covered by my shirt, but I will know it is there. It will be a reminder that I am fortunate to live in a time when medical technology can correct some problems and not others. We have made medical progress since my dad's death, now we need to find a cause and cure for dysautonomia.

INDEPENDENCE

Independence Day 2014: I went with my family to fireworks festivities for the first time in several years. As I gazed up at the sky, breathed in the fresh air, and watched the beautiful show I marveled at life and freedom. My 11-year-old glanced at me often with a huge smile; and if I could read his mind, I am certain it would say he was happy to have mom with him. Late in the show we held hands and my husband reached for the other, as our daughter rested on his shoulder. It was a peaceful, celebratory evening.

Independence - able to take care of oneself without outside help. Synonyms include

**self-dependent, self-reliant, autonomous, re-
silient, strong.**

Independence is a tricky concept. There are always choices to make in this chronic illness journey. I want to believe I am independent, self-reliant, and strong. Choices come with consequences. Victories produce deficits. The fireworks display was spectacular but came with an ocular migraine and exhaustion the following day. Coincidence? Probably not.

Independence - it is what we most want but dysautonomia takes some of it away. There are doctors, medicines, and people we must depend upon for help. We can't do what we want when we want as there are consequences to our actions. Energy is a premium which when used is gone until it decides to return. There is no logic to the energy/currency dilemma.

It is a very thin/fine line between dependence and independence. It is a balancing act that becomes cloudy. Sometimes I believe I'm independent and my body revolts and I must depend on others for assistance. It may be as simple as getting me a drink from the refrigerator or driving to a doctor's appointment. I don't enjoy seeking help from others as I am stubborn and like to be self-reliant.

It is ironic that as early as we can remember we struggle for independence, but in an instant life can change and that freedom can be altered. Independence is a gift and privilege, something to be celebrated. When it is taken from us the results are startling.

<u>BROKEN</u>

Broken - fractured or damaged and no longer in one piece or working order. Having given up all hope, despairing.

I have noticed my limitations more lately. Perhaps it is because I have stretched my body extensively - attending two funerals in the last three weeks; making sure I am ready for an upcoming charity ride; helping the kids with end-of-the year activities and carting my daughter to physical therapy (PT) now that she had her fourth knee surgery.

Of course, there are the added surprises of ocular migraines, which come without warning and stop everything in their way. I am flattened and afterwards left exhausted, nauseous and in pain.

Today I sit in a PT waiting room with legs crossed over my lap. I am the only one sitting this way and some might think I am just relaxed. I may or may not be relaxed. I must keep my legs up as otherwise sitting will cause blood pooling, varying blood pressure and elevated pulse.

I am annoyed when someone mentions how relaxed I look, but I usually just smile. I find it amazing and frustrating that the simple act of sitting or standing can cause such problems. I could just stay home and recline but then I would not be living.

I persevere but wish I had a better functioning body.

I have learned how to accommodate myself regardless of the situation. At my daughter's athletic program I ended up third from the aisle in the crammed row with nowhere for my feet to go but down. I knew the only solution was to move up a few rows and sit alone on the end. I did not expect my husband and daughter to join me, but I was a bit frustrated. I stayed healthy enough to sit for two hours but sitting alone was the tradeoff.

I guess it is all about trade-offs. I can't do what I once did; energy is not there nor is the body's ability to compensate. I mostly accept this, however once in a while I get stuck, frustrated, angry. I would love a day in which my body did not remind me it is broken.

INVISIBLE

We recently recognized Invisible Illness Week, a time to celebrate and raise awareness of those dealing with medical conditions that are not visible to others.

Invisible - unable to be seen, not visible. Ignored or not taken into consideration.

Invisible - that is a difficult word to digest. Those dealing with chronic or long-term illness have a difficult enough time handling the ramifications of such illnesses. Can you imagine being ignored by others?

It is hard to comprehend but many have been ignored or their illnesses minimized. I have heard more times than I can count "you look so good." It is a confusing statement as one wonders if that is a compliment or rather a way for others to say "y'know you look too healthy to be sick, it can't be that bad."

I could give examples of feeling minimized, but I won't.

When it happens, I feel invisible, hidden and ignored. I don't like attention; there are times I would like to fade in the background. And that's the paradox because these illnesses make us feel invisible sometimes, yet we crave to be treated normally.

One of the best things someone did for me since being diagnosed is treat me like a person, not an illness. A former colleague hugged me when I saw him, said how are you doing, how are your kids, and then listened until I asked the same of him.

Listening is a great validator. It is easy, free and produces amazing results.

God listens and is a constant support to those in need. Remember we are surrounded by this love always and must share love with others.

CONFIDENCE MY BODY WILL REVOLT

Confidence - reliance on one's circumstances; a certainty; a belief that one will act in the proper way.

When I look at that definition I grimace. At times, my body does not emit confidence. I am sure my blood pressure could be anywhere on the spectrum; my hands may turn purple; and a myriad of other things could happen. But am I certain that I can rely on my body when I need to for big events? Hardly.

Here is the interesting spin to this uncertainty. I don't get as nervous or scared about whether my body will perform the way I want it to. Rather I prepare the best I can for an event. In my situation it means pacing activities, drinking fluids (perhaps scheduling intravenous fluids around an event), praying, exercising, eating the best I can and resting. I also try to enter a situation with a plan of where to go if I need to exit quickly for some reason. I then enjoy the experience; marvel at what I am doing, whom I am with and what is occurring. I don't expect the experience to be flawless - symptoms will occur- but hopefully I will manage and if not I usually know how to handle such.

Of course, there is sadness of what I cannot do; some days the word chronic becomes overwhelming; but more so I try to relish the good.

Confidence can certainly be shaken. People with chronic illness exhibit great courage and endurance. And with God all things are possible.

CHRONIC IS A NEVER-ENDING EXPERIENCE

Chronic - persisting for a long time or constantly recurring. Chronic contrasts with acute.

Chronic illness is an accurate definition of an ongoing medical problem. Here are some thoughts on having a chronic illness in no relevant order:

1. Each day is unpredictable, which is both exciting and annoying. I never know what my body will do. I can be enjoying a time out at Starbucks and suddenly will need to elevate my feet, run to a

bathroom or lie flat. Or perhaps an outing will be uneventful, and I will have fun. Since I never know the outcome, the best thing to do is enjoy the good moments while they occur.

2. There is a bit too much quiet time in my life. Without a career there are parts of the day that become too quiet. This is when thoughts can turn sad, lonely and hopeless. It is okay to feel this way, but the key is to find balance. I know when I do things during the day, even little things, I feel more hope filled.

3. Chronic means long. This illness is a challenge and unless a miracle changes things it is not going to end. The illness stays in my mind, a constant reminder of what is different in life. It brings with it both sadness and joy. If I let my thoughts get too far into the future things will get hopeless; so that is not an option.

4. People have a difficult time understanding chronic illness unless they live with it. Some will ask ridiculous questions and even become jealous because I don't work anymore. They have no idea the amount of energy it takes to remain upright and never will, no matter how many times it is explained. It is not worth the effort.

5. Energy is currency. Once it is expended it may not come back for a while. Even sleep may not restore energy. For this reason, people dealing with chronic conditions have to choose very carefully what to

do and not do. Sometimes it may not make sense how we can do one thing but not another. But without living in our bodies, it is best not to judge us as people have no idea of all the variables.

6. Every day I feel unwell at some point, but I don't care most of the time. What I care more about is life and living it the best I can. When you see me, instead of asking me how I am, what do I do all day or saying I look so good, just treat me like you treat everyone else. That will help me to feel somewhat normal. Because honestly there is not much normal about taking upwards of 25 medicines and vitamins daily, getting weekly IV saline at home, having several doctors, a pacemaker and being retired at 49.

7. I get angry sometimes and would like to throw my IV pole out the window and pretend my body worked normally. I would like to get in my car and drive the four hours to Cleveland by myself to visit a friend; go shopping all day; take a 15- mile bike ride; never see another needle; eat a regular meal at a leisurely pace at a restaurant after attending a Buffalo Sabres' game; go for an hour walk at a local park with steep hills and many other things. But right now, those things are no longer in the realm of possibility. I find other things to do and remember that I am alive, blessed and continue to try each day to embrace life.

It is not easy, but life is not always easy.

FIVE YEARS LATER PACEMAKER GETS A NAME

It took five years to find but it was worth the wait. When my daughter asked today if I had a name, Blossom quickly popped into my head. And it fits.

Blossom - a peak period or state of development. To bloom.

Five years ago my life began to blossom after being dulled by dysautonomia. That Wednesday afternoon, Oct. 9, Dr. Blair Grubb of the University of Toledo Medical Center implanted a pacemaker which immediately eliminated bradycardia, or a heartbeat under 60 beats per minute. This has allowed me more stamina and ability to do more things each day.

In five years, the pacemaker has provided approximately 36,792,000 heartbeats that has been impossible beforehand. Today I celebrated, taking in a beautiful eight-mile bike ride. The original plan was to attend church and then conquer the hill that eight years prior had forced me off my bike; an indication that something was medically wrong. But yesterday was physically difficult. After biking seven miles I had to jump off the bike to avert puking. To avoid the risk of being stranded too far from home today, I chose a different route.

Today I felt fabulous. I prayed while pedaling and marveled at my ability to bike despite dysautonomia. And I wondered had more technology been available in 1976 would my father gotten a pacemaker and lived longer than 48 years. Had he been born a few decades later he may have had a better chance at life. But of course, that was not the case and despite losing him too early to a massive heart attack I am so thankful for his love and guidance throughout my life.

I have been fortunate to have met an amazing cardiologist who has helped me to gain health. He has allowed me to bloom; experience life again and to realize life has so many blessings.

I have about 36.8 million additional beats to use until Blossom will need changing. I hope to have more bike rides and adventures. I know this medical road will not always be easy but with a pacemaker, God and my family and friends I will persevere.

The steadfast love of the Lord never ceases,

his mercies never come to an end;

they are new every morning;

   great is thy faithfulness.

"The Lord is my portion," says my soul,

   "therefore, I will hope in him."

(Lamentations 3:22-24).

WE NEED A TOOLBOX TO COPE WITH ILLNESS

Toolbox - a container in which you keep and carry small tools, especially those used in the house or for repairing a car.

Carpenters, mechanics and construction workers use toolboxes. But I think all people could use a toolbox.

What's in your toolbox?

I'm reminded of this question and think back to when I taught conflict resolution skills to fourth graders at school. First, we read a story about two neighbors fighting over a piece of property. Eventually the students devised peaceful solution; building a friendship bridge to connect the properties.

Students were then directed to construct a paper toolbox and tools.

Tools - something (such as an instrument or apparatus) used in performing an operation or necessary in the practice of a vocation or profession, a means to an end.

Some drew the typical hammer and nails but then were challenged to find other objects for the box. The objects would be things in their metaphoric box which could help them in life to handle conflicts and relationships in general.

While exercising recently, I realized I need to update my own toolbox and dust of the neglected items. Because two weeks of ups and downs with my health leave me worried that I will miss upcoming events .

I need to dust off my tools and develop more. I also need to find the enthusiasm to do this as trying to be well is a daunting task at times. Here are some of my toolbox items.

- Exercise
- Prayer
- Music

- Writing
- Reading
- Family and friends
- Church
- Dogs
- Husband
- Grace for when I'm not feeling well or need to rest
- Patience with myself
- Hope that tomorrow will be better
- Perseverance to continue to try to have good days

Tools are helpful if we use them.

This is a reminder I need today.

THINGS WE CAN STILL DO TO ENJOY LIFE

Despite our physical limitations there are still things we can enjoy. These may include:

- Attend a Cleveland Orchestra concert.
- Visit Emerald Necklace (A park system around greater Cleveland).
- Have ice cream contests (for our anniversary, we went to several ice cream places to decide which were our favorites).
- Provide fairy godmother surprises - giving other's cards, small gifts and surprises out of the blue.
- Learn new skills.
- Develop an artistic side.
- Volunteer.

- Pray.
- Plant new vegetables yearly.
- Exercise. Start slow and work up your endurance. Dysautonomia specialists often recommend using a recumbent bike and rowing machine, and swimming. Weight training can also be helpful.
- Select new colors in plants.
- Read classics. My discerning quest is: "what wisdom has survived for generations?"
- Ask "how have you used the gifts you were given to help others?" Helping others is empowering.
- While we may not be able to travel to other continents, we can still enjoy people's travel stories.
- Crochet, knit or do other art forms.
- Cook.
- Read; join a book club, or a library reading club. Try a new author.
- Whittle down your outfits to only what you love. Discern your best color.
- Find you favorite unscented lotion. Play with make-up.
- Laugh.
- Figure out who are your favorite classical, country, blues, and rock musicians. For example, make March music month. Try different artists each week. No foolin' by April 1, you will have preferences.

- Over time, a joy pattern evolved. My isolated suffering "God help me" moments helped to decipher what is important and what can be eliminated. Love always wins.

DIARY QUESTIONS

What is in your toolbox and what additional items could you put into it?

Do you have any words that resonate with you and if so, what are they and why?

How do you enjoy yourself when you experience occasional wellness?

How do you deal with the fact that your chronic illness does not currently have a cure?

What do you do to help other people, or what could you do to help someone who lives with a chronic condition?

Chapter eight: Reflections...

"Be who you are, and be that well."
—St. Francis de Sales

"If your actions inspire others to dream more, learn more, do more, become more, you are a leader."
—John Quincy Adams

"Nothing can stop God's plan for your life."
—Isaiah 14;27

Living with dysautonomia or any chronic condition can feel overwhelming. There are opportunities, also, that may come our way. I had an amazing privilege through Dysautonomia International of honoring my cardiologist with physician of the year in 2015. The following is the nomination of Dr. Blair Grubb.

DYSAUTONOMIA INTL. DOCTOR OF THE YEAR

You hear his name, see it throughout the research on dysautonomia and expect a giant when you finally meet him. And when I say finally, I mean finally because it is not easy to secure an appointment with this autonomic specialist.

In fact, I waited 16 months before trekking the 300-miles each way to Toledo, Ohio for an appointment with Dr. Blair Grubb at the University of Toledo Heart and Vascular Center.

I first met Dr. Grubb in the summer of 2012 and travel two-three times a year for follow-up appointments.

After hearing so much about this man, I did not know what to expect. From what I understood, he was one of the experts in the field _ of which unfortunately there are few. In my mind he held a key to my health, my destiny. I prayed and hoped he would help me; give me a better quality of life. I had been referred to him by a doctor who basically minimized my symptoms despite the fact I had to retire early from my beloved job as an elementary school counselor. Dysautonomia was robbing me of my ability to sit upright and think, producing crazy symptoms, taking away my normal life. Would this man dismiss me like the other cardiologist had or would he help?

If you have met Dr. Blair Grubb, you know the answers to these questions? He walked into the examining room and greeted my husband and me with a warm handshake and smile. He listened, explained the autonomic nervous system to us, examined me, and gave answers and hope that we would -together- find a treatment plan that gave me a better quality of life. And he hugged me and told me to be well -something he does at every visit.

As our patient/doctor relationship grew, Dr. Grubb began greeting me with a welcome smile and embrace. He sits down and listens and then decides what the treatment options are.

Dr. Grubb improved my quality of life tremendously in Oct. 2013 when he implanted a BIOTRONIK EVIA pacemaker. This pacemaker works well with dysautonomia patients who have bradycardia as it responds to both heart rate and blood pressure. I cannot explain the mechanics of this but know that Dr. Grubb was a leading cardiologist to first use this pacer. After a failed attempt at raising my heart rate through Adderall, he recommended in August 2013 that we implant the pacemaker sooner, rather than later, as I was operating at 40-50 beats per minute and it was affecting the quality of my life.

I spent eight weeks, from the time I found out about the surgery, until the actual date, worried. During this time, I made several calls to Dr. Grubb's office and at one point he spent about 30 minutes on the telephone answering my questions. I knew I was in good hands prior to that phone call but afterwards felt more at ease. Dr. Grubb, you see, treats patients from all over the world; is usually behind schedule and works long into the evening to see everyone. He spends as much time as necessary to see each patient in the clinic, but yet he did not rush me on the telephone. And when I asked him if he plays music in his operating room (yes) and has fun doing surgeries (yes) I knew I was in good hands.

My surgery went well but after the BIOTRONIK representative set my pacemaker rate much higher than I agreed upon or could handle the morning after surgery, my nurse intervened. Dr. Grubb personally found me in the x-ray department and reassured me the pacer would be reset to a lower rate. It was taken care of immediately.

Despite the fact this man is pulled in so many directions, Dr. Grubb puts his patients' wellbeing first, as this example and many others show.

At a follow-up a few weeks later; and on subsequent visits, Dr. Grubb has ended his conversations the same way. He has hugged me, told me to "be well," and "live."

Live - to exhibit vigor, gusto or enthusiasm.

Live life to the fullest: to experience firsthand.

Since meeting Dr. Grubb, I wear a bracelet on my left arm. It reads "Live." It is a reminder to take each day as it comes; but also, to try to live in the present; to savior every moment, enjoy each blessing.

Dysautonomia is still a part of my life. I struggle with daily symptoms. But I do my best to live, and my quality of life is improved. Having 62 beats per minutes is a beautiful thing that makes me feel a bit stronger. It has allowed me to get back on my beloved road bike. And while I can't ride as far, I completed a 10-mile charity event for cancer research this past June and raised $1700. This is something I had not been able to do since being diagnosed in

2010. Biking is trickier and I must stop, stretch my legs out, drink fluids and wait a bit before finishing up some rides. But that is ok, at least I can ride.

I give all the credit for this regained health to God first and then Dr. Grubb.

CONQUERING HILL THAT BEGAN THIS JOURNEY

I rode 12.2 miles on my bike.

There are two reasons this is a huge event. First, I have not ridden this far since 2009.

And second, I conquered a hill that had not been attempted since summer, 2010. That summer day I finished biking this exact hill but had to dive abruptly off my bike to the grass. My heart screamed, head pounded, and eyes were hazy. This was the first of three times I nearly passed out while biking; and it was clear that my body was betraying me. I now know that these near faints were signs of dysautonomia.

For the last few months, I had been thinking of trying to bike this hill again, now that a pacemaker beats inside of me. Today was the day. After biking four miles to the road, I stopped briefly for a drink and to catch my breath. Then I was off, pedaling in low gear up the steep climb. Halfway up, I stopped again, caught my breath and continued.

My heart was pounding as I reached the top. I felt a bit like puking but I was alive and fighting back from this disorder that has robbed me and others of so much. It was a beautiful, 70-plus degree November day, and I had just conquered my fear of riding up that hill again.

I am tired, but it is a good tired knowing I pushed my body and won. It is a liberating feeling.

While riding this morning I swore several times at the hill. Really, though, it was me yelling at this disorder. I won't let it win, despite best efforts. It grabs and holds on tightly. But I am strong and am determined to live my best life despite dysautonomia.

LOSS OF DOCTOR PRODUCES UNCERTAINTY

I said goodbye to my primary care doctor. He is moving south to operate a satellite office of a major hospital. It was an opportunity too good to pass. I am genuinely happy for him; but with this change comes apprehension for me.

People dealing with chronic conditions know that when we find a competent, caring doctor we hold on tightly to them.

I have known Dr. Deberny for 21 years, fresh out of medical school. I saw several physicians in the practice at that time, but on December 30, 2010 he became my primary doctor. It was my 22nd wedding anniversary. I had suffered with migraines and dizziness all of December and ended up with this doctor on my second sick visit in four days. After determining I was severely dehydrated, he pumped two bags of fluids into me and remarkably I felt better. This was my first of many experiences with intravenous therapy.

The appointment was pivotal as he put me on a three-week sick leave. We did not know then that my autonomic nervous system was misfiring. In subsequent months, as my health spiraled downward, this doctor never lost hope of helping me. In fact, he apologized early on for not knowing what was wrong; how to treat me.

We persevered together. Since that day, I have had 56 office visits. Of that number 48 were with him.

Dr. Deberny stuck with me from the beginning; learned more about dysautonomia than he ever probably wanted to; listened; reassured when I was fearful and encouraged me to get a pacemaker. And we talked about God.

I am leery about finding a new doctor; but I will do two things to hopefully gain another amazing primary care physician. I will meet several doctors and see how they operate; and I will trust God to lead me to the proper provider. Just like He did so many years ago.

UNDERSTANDING AND HELPING

Living with someone who has a chronic illness can be difficult. Here are a few suggestions of ways to handle such:

- Remember we are still the same person whom you love; we just may have different stripes. Maybe we cannot do the same things we did before illness, but we are still us.

- Understand our diagnosis. You don't have to study dysautonomia 101 but have a general idea of what it does to our bodies. Believe us when we tell you of medical symptoms, even if we outwardly look healthy.

- Realize that some of the things we do we have no control over. We can't control when our vital signs go haywire, causing fog and other symptoms. Understand we are trying to function the best we can.

- We don't need you to fix our problems; rather we just need support. This could be as simple as guiding us out of a crowded store that has caused sensory overload; to getting us a drink and blanket when we need to recline.

- Find new things to enjoy with us. Maybe we can't get out to dinner or a movie, but can do takeout and Netflix.

- Spend time with us. Our day can become lonely and human contact is comforting.

- Talk to someone about our situation. It is stressful knowing you are the healthier one, the one who must carry a heavier load. Talk to a friend, counselor, spiritual advisor, anyone you trust. Share some of the stress, it will unburden you a bit.

- Know that we try every day to live our best life. Sitting upright and standing are challenging to our bodies. This takes massive energy even though we may look healthy. Understand we are not lazy; rather our bodies are so skewed we need to rest at times.

- Realize we are blessed. We are blessed in our

relationships with others. And many of us cherish the tinniest thing that much more. Getting out for a bit, seeing friends, engaging with others are activities we relish when we can do them.

- Know our stamina has been greatly reduced. Once we have reached our limit, we are done. We must rest, we have no option, no choice. It is crucial.

- We appreciate those who stay despite our illness. Many have left, perhaps afraid they would "catch" it.

TIDBITS/RESOURCES

Below is a list of information/products which may be helpful in dealing with autonomic dysfunction.

- Dysautonomia International <u>dysautonomiainternational.org</u> - provides vast information and support. Also provides research money to medical personnel to study dysautonomia and best practices for treatment.

- Antigravity chairs. You can put your feet higher than your heart. Purchase a portable one.

- Handicapped parking permit. This hangtag will help you park closer and conserve precious energy walking in the parking lot, or in the store. Each state does the application process a bit differently, but basically you fill out an application and have your doctor sign off. It is then submitted to the proper authority (could be your motor vehicle bureau or town government) where you will get the tag. Keep in safe place and affix to mirror when you park.

- Cooling cloth; keep in the refrigerator during the summer. It feels great against forehead or back of neck, when you have that self-igniting feeling.
- Humor. This diagnosis is absurd, we need to laugh often.
- Flannel blankets and sweaters for changing temperatures.
- Nabee compression socks - can be ordered online.
- Four wheeled walkers, with a basket in the seat.
- Medical identification band; this will give you and your family security when you venture outside the home.
- List of your diagnoses, medications, doctors and emergency contacts in your wallet or purse. Also place on your refrigerator in case you need to call emergency medical people to your home.
- Journal, separators for labs/ testing/ and antidotal journal entries. Keep medical records organized and updated.
- NUUN tablets: flavored, electrolyte enhanced tablets, found in sporting good stores and online.
- NormaLYTE, high sodium, powdered drink. Found online and in limited stores.
- Pill sorter. These will save so much time and will help you remember to take medications.
- Keep medication bottles in a secure, safe box, away from reach of kids and animals.

- Amazon.com - can purchase hydration supplies, compression clothing, food, books and gifts.
- Electric blankets are warm and cozy, especially during cold months.
- Shower chairs, mats and bars provide safety.
- Pretzels with peanut butter, protein shakes, cheese sticks and nuts.
- Mints for nausea. I like ginger mints from Trader Joe's.
- I-Pad, Kindle or another tablet. This can be used to listen to music, write, watch television, play games, read and connect with others on the internet. Have an extra charger on hand.
- Body wash - can be used for quicker showers.
- Car starter to warm or cool car prior to driving.
- Kitchen stool for cooking and sea salt ready to ingest at any time.
- Ammonia sticks taped on mirror.
- Cell phone and chargers.
- TheMighty.com - internet site that provides stories/ information on many conditions.

DIARY QUESTIONS

What advice would you give family and friends recently diagnosed with a chronic illness?

Do you wish people knew about chronic illness?

What are three of your strengths?

What is a resource you discovered which has been helpful in dealing with medical condition(s)?

EPILOGUE

The roller coaster ride of dysautonomia continues for Sharon and I since this book was completed. We both have faced additional health challenges that have tested both our faith and bodies. We continue to persevere despite these stressors.

Sharon has added the diagnosis of idiopathic anaphylaxis with Kounis syndrome. Her team believes that having the measles as a child resulted in Sharon's immune and autonomic nervous systems being damaged. She also had childhood evidence of syncope and other symptoms. Under the dysautonomia umbrella she has scoliosis, Sjogren's syndrome, hypothyroidism and mast cell activation disorder.

Sharon has been admitted to the ICU several times after experiencing anaphylactic episodes. Her heart enzymes increased and thankfully her doctors ruled out heart attack. She has added an amazing cardiologist to her medical team.

Despite this precarious health, Sharon chooses to live each day to the fullest. She bakes for a local food shelter, crochets dolls and blankets for different causes and is a self-proclaimed Fairy Godmother - trying to bring joy to those she cares about in unexpected ways. It is not unusual for me to receive a random card/package from Sharon which always brightens my day. And I am sure I am one of many people who are on the end of her generosity.

I have added Sjogren's syndrome, hypothyroid, mitochondrial myopathy, small fibre neuropathy and several food intolerances/allergies to my list of medical issues. I've also dealt with pancreatitis -which may be tied to my other health issues. This last problem has left me scrambling to figure out what I can eat. Thankfully eliminating many foods from my diet has improved digestion and reduced pain.

In November, 2022 I had a new pacemaker - a BIOTRONIK Edora implanted. It is similar to the previous pacer but is MRI compatible. This will be helpful if I need diagnostic tests.

I also experienced a two-month bout with depression. I believe depression was a culmination of an added diagnosis, change in medication and mounting grief from the many losses chronic illness present. I am unaccustomed to such hopeless feelings and sought the help of my husband, a few close friends (including Sharon), my counselor and God to assist me in climbing out of this pit. I hope to never experience depression again but am realistic in knowing that medical stressors can be a cause of such. I am a firm believer in counseling to deal with the varied losses and challenges of chronic conditions. I also have been fortunate to have regained my primary care doctor. He did not like his new out-of-state position so came back to his previous practice. Thankfully I had stayed with the practice, seeing a different doctor, so easily switched back to him.

In 2020 I dealt with a two-week illness we believe was COVID 19 (testing was not available at that time). Thankfully I was not hospitalized but the aftereffects of the illness including inflammation throughout my body, the necessity for two inhalers daily for 16 months and a lung CT-scan that showed ground glass cluster. I also had a change in my aorta and wall thickening that both my cardiologist and immunologist believe may be an after-effect of the illness. At this point, I must get a CT-scan regularly to monitor the situation. I have been told that the amount of biking I did may have helped me to recover better from this illness.

Living with chronic illness is difficult. But it is amazing how we learn to advocate for our own health and make connections with other people also dealing with chronic conditions. When we meet others like us, there is an instant bond and common understanding. This is very validating.

Sharon and I have learned many things during our 12-year-friendship. These include:

Try to find the humor in the situation.

Be your own advocate. Know as much as you can about your medical situation (without becoming compulsive) so you can receive the best possible treatment.

Every person's body reacts differently; what may work for one person may not work for the next.

A tiny slice of denial is healthy. Realize that you have a

condition but don't become that illness. Try to do things and when your body revolts rest.

Pacing is crucial. Plan out how you will expend energy but realize your plans can go haywire if your body does not cooperate. (This is super difficult for me to practice).

Don't become obsessed with blood pressure readings or other medical facts. If you need to take your blood pressure to gather information or on doctor's orders, go ahead. But don't become compulsive.

Gauge what you can do based on how you feel. If you have a little more energy one day perhaps do something you enjoy. Understand the activity may deplete energy, but hopefully the activity is worth the effort.

Exercise is very important both physically and emotionally. It may also reduce pain. Seek medical advice before starting an exercise plan and understand building your stamina is a long process.

Nurture your relationships. Stress is a byproduct of our illnesses; make sure to take time to talk with and listen to loved ones.

There is a lot we cannot control; yet there is much we can. This includes our thoughts and taking steps to manage our conditions. It is not an easy process, but we must persevere the best we can.

It is vital to take medications as scheduled and drink the prescribed fluid amount necessary to help our bodies. Invest in a weekly pill organizer. This will save time and assist in keeping track of medications.

Remember it is alright to become angry when knocked

down with another problem, symptom or diagnosis. But don't stay angry. Own it, deal with it (and the sadness, frustration, confusion...that comes with it) and move on. Sharon and I typically get downright mad for a week or less, then try to get back to our emotional baseline.

Find a support system that works for you. Counselors, physical therapists, yoga instructors, chiropractors, clergy and others can be of assistance.

Ask for help. Some churches provide meals when people are in medical crises or experiencing other problems. When friends ask if they can help, tell them specifically what you need. Whether it's company, a meal or a ride to an appointment, no one can read our minds. Honesty is appreciated.

We are strong. We endure a lot of things on this medical ride. Each day offers new opportunities to improve. Finding what helps us function better and developing a routine is productive.

If your doctor wants to try a new medication, voice concerns and weigh the benefits against the possible side effects. Ask all the questions you need to make an informed decision. It is often helpful to give a medication a try for two-three weeks to really see how it works on your body. Of course, if side effects are serious from the beginning, let your doctor know immediately so the doctor can advise you of how to titrate off the medications. Do not just stop a medication without medical advice.

Remind your doctor, if applicable, that the smallest dose of a medication is often the best dose to start with as we are often very sensitive to medications.

Don't lose yourself in this process. There is little that is easy about living with dysautonomia and other chronic conditions. But we need to remember who we are; our joys; our accomplishments. We are not our diagnosis and must work to not be seen as such.

Educate yourself on your diagnoses; but use valid sites and top research to get information. Dysautonomia International has great resources and is a medically valid site.

Try not to get too down on yourself. This is a difficult life living with chronic illness. Give yourself the grace to make mistakes but keep trying. If you have a difficult day or two or three, that is ok. Just persevere. Try to use positive self-talk if you get stuck in a negative rut.

Laugh.

Eat chocolate.

God bless you on your journey.
2023.

Made in the USA
Middletown, DE
12 May 2023

29797199R00149